DATE DUE

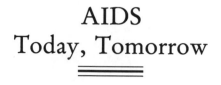

AIDS
Today, Tomorrow

AIDS
Today, Tomorrow

═══════

An Introduction to the
HIV Epidemic in America

ROBERT SEARLES WALKER

Humanities Press International, Inc.
New Jersey and London

First published 1991 by Humanities Press International, Inc.
Atlantic Highlands, New Jersey 07716, and
3 Henrietta Street, London WC2E 8LU

© Robert S. Walker, 1991

Library of Congress Cataloging-in-Publication Data
Walker, Robert Searles, 1930–
    AIDS—today, tomorrow : an introduction to the HIV epidemic in
America / Robert Searles Walker.
      p.   cm.
    Includes bibliographical references and index.
    ISBN 0–391–03719–6. — ISBN 0–391–03712–9 (pbk.)
    1. AIDS (Disease)—United States.   I. Title.
RC607.A26W35   1991
362.1'9697'9200973—dc20   91–7902
                                                                  CIP

British Cataloguing in Publication Data
Walker, Robert Searles
    AIDS : today, tomorrow.
    I. Title
    362.1042

    ISBN 0391037196
    ISBN 0391037129 (paperback)

Printed in the United States of America

Contents

List of Illustrations

List of Tables

Preface

Five years ago I lost the first of many friends to AIDS. During the hours of visiting at the hospital, I tried to understand what was happening, to make some sense of it. Why should he have been so afflicted at so young an age, only 27? How was it that in medically advanced America, there was no effective treatment, much less a cure? Like most Americans I grew up believing that we could deal effectively with all but the rarest ailments. But AIDS was becoming increasingly common, and it targeted youth—the age group that enrolled in my classes. By 1986 the Human Immunodeficiency Virus had already infected 1 out of every 30 American men between the ages of 20 and 50. My friend's death led to a personal research effort as I sought answers.

In 1987 I was obliged to organize my general understanding of the epidemic. Biology Professor Richard Siegel (University of California at Los Angeles) invited me to give some lectures on the political and social aspects of the epidemic. Dr. Siegel was a pioneer in the development of general education courses on sexually transmitted diseases. His efforts in this field were, like mine, a personal response, but of a different sort. His children asked him why his college was not offering any general courses on a topic of increasing interest to those in their sexually active age group. They definitely wanted to know about AIDS, and not as a problem of retrovirology, but as a problem confronting their lives. Dr. Siegel responded with an excellent and successful course at UCLA. In the process of preparing my lectures for that course, the themes of this book began to emerge. Overall, it is the product of trying to make sense out of the tidal wave of death that was beginning to break over the nation, threatening my children, my students, and my friends.

The spread of the virus is uneven, both globally and within the United States. However, it will gradually spread everywhere. While the focus of this book is on the national picture, I have used data from Texas, including my city of San Antonio. I hope thereby to encourage readers to look to their own areas, their state and city health agencies, their communities for parallels and comparisons. There is a strong tendency to shrug off the agonies and lessons of New York City and San Francisco as irrelevant to "our town." But they definitely are relevant! It is just a matter of time. The

1990 data indicated that the virus was beginning to spread into our smaller cities and rural areas, and an average of 2,000+ new cases were being recorded monthly.

As the AIDS epidemic grows it will capture an increasing share of the nation's attention and resources. More people will be compelled to confront it intellectually and emotionally. A total of 450,000 cases is projected for 1993. If you assume that each Person with AIDS (PWA) relates to just four other people—family and friends—then the total intimately affected by the epidemic equals roughly 10% of our population. Even those not directly and personally affected will feel the impact as taxes, lost productivity, and other costs begin to mount. And the epidemic is in its early, not late, stages.

Willingly or otherwise, millions of people will be thinking about AIDS. The range of issues raised by the epidemic is extraordinary—from simple problems (avoiding infection), through tangled ones (the political difficulties of insuring catastrophic health care), to the downright baffling (the complexities of vaccine development). It is my hope that this study, by viewing the epidemic from many different perspectives, will help concerned individuals to think about the problems raised by AIDS for themselves, their communities, their nation, and their world. Think about AIDS we must, for it is idle fantasy to imagine that any of us will be left untouched by the greatest biologic scourge of our time.

This is a brief introductory work. Like all of its kind, it must oversimplify, sometimes embarrassingly so. The epidemic is an exceptionally complex phenomenon in all its manifestations, from the nature of the virus itself to the epidemic's impact on our culture. In all cases I have tried to point the reader to more extensive treatments of whatever topic the text takes up. For example, Chapter 2 renders a very generalized, elementary account of the life cycle of the virus, but the reader will find in the endnotes reference to more complex and comprehensive descriptions up to and including those from molecular biology and virology. I would have my readers regard each of the chapters as a door through which they can pass in order to view in greater detail, if they wish, some aspect of this far-reaching phenomenon.

I would like to thank my friend Esta Wolfram for her generous and significant assistance, both in collecting data and in editing the text. Many thanks are due also to Dorothy Williams, as well as other staff of the Trinity University Library, for various kinds of freely given help, from copy reading to searches. My research was enriched by a steady stream of medical bulletins and journals fed me by Major Robert Munson, M.D. (USAF), for which I am grateful. I was also able to draw upon the resources of the San Antonio AIDS Foundation and the wide-ranging knowledge of its president, Papa Bear. None of those people can be held accountable for the shortcomings of this book, but all can claim some credit for its virtues.

Finally to my wife, Joyce, my deepest gratitude, not only for her constant encouragement and constructive comments as this work progressed, but also for her tolerance and care of a moody, withdrawn, and distracted author.

Trinity University
San Antonio, Texas

1

===

AIDS: Plague or Epidemic? What's in a Word?

In 1976 Professor William McNeill published a challenging and provocative book, *Plagues and Peoples*, that explored the impact of epidemics in history. In his conclusion, he noted the progress made in containing such historic killers as the bubonic plague, smallpox, and cholera, but cautioned his readers to remember that the biologic agents of epidemics are always with us; they never just go away. Medicines and public health measures may keep them at bay, but none have been eradicated. Further, he reminded:

> it is always possible that some hitherto obscure parasitic organism may escape its accustomed ecological niche and expose the dense human populations that have become so conspicuous a feature of earth to some fresh and perchance devastating mortality.[1]

You and I are living out the scholar's careful reservation. Events force us to face the truth that we are in the beginning throes of a major world epidemic attributable to a "hitherto obscure parasitic organism," the human immunodeficiency virus (HIV). We must recapture a knowledge our ancestors knew well, namely that epidemics are natural, recurring events, like earthquakes. The acquired immunodeficiency syndrome (AIDS) caused by HIV is not the first, nor will it be the last epidemic to afflict humanity. It is but one of the inescapable hazards that are part of life and death on the planet Earth.

The AIDS epidemic is the "devastating mortality" that Professor McNeill's words foreshadowed. It is sometimes referred to as a "plague" and sometimes as an "epidemic" in sermons, media accounts, and general

---

This chapter is based on a series of lectures delivered in January 1988 to the Sexually Transmitted Diseases class at the University of California at Los Angeles.

conversation. Should the semantics make a difference; are the terms syn-
onymous? What's in a word?

Words, our choice of words, matter enormously. Words denote the
objects or ideas that we are trying to convey. They also carry a hidden
baggage of emotion and prejudice that quietly but decisively direct action. A
word can be like the proverbial iceberg, nine-tenths underwater, unseen, and
ten times more deadly for that![2] So many illustrations of this come to mind
that it is hard to choose. Consider the words that we have stricken from the
acceptable public vocabulary in only the last 25 years—"nigger," "kike,"
"wop," "dumb broad," "spic," and (almost, but not quite) "queer." We are
in the process of excising these words from our public speech because they
co-opt thinking rather than promote it, they cloud rather than clarify debate,
and they inflame emotions rather than engage the mind. Recently there have
been heated debates in church groups about whether references to "God the
Father" should be changed to gender-neutral terms like "Holy Spirit."
Behind the semantic issue are the deeper ones relating to our perception of
deity and of ourselves, issues about which our species has always fought
with both ballots and bullets.

How do such considerations apply to choosing a designation for
AIDS—"plague" or "epidemic"? All the great mortalities of the past were
known by one or the other term. For example, the devastation caused by
Yersinia pestis has always been called the bubonic plague, while the havoc
wrought by *Vibrio cholerae* is referred to as a cholera epidemic. We speak of
a "plague" of locusts, but an "epidemic" of measles. The ancient curse is: "A
plague on both your houses!"—never "an epidemic." For AIDS, the em-
phatic choice must be "epidemic." AIDS is an *epidemic*, not a plague.

Why? What's in a word? Is it much ado about nothing? AIDS was quickly
labeled a plague, although previous twentieth century visitations (cholera in
1900, Spanish flu in 1918, and infantile paralysis) were all called epidemics. Is
it just a matter of contemporary versus traditional usage? No, not really. The
truly classic words used to name these terrible events were "pestilence" or
"mortality." Perhaps we distinguish between plagues and epidemics based
on their relative prowess as killers. There is, after all, a sense hovering
around the word "plague" that suggests something extraordinarily deadly
and fearsome. But truthfully, it requires a worst-case, long-term scenario for
AIDS to match past mortalities. Cholera killed 7 million in the first 20 years
of this century and struck again in 1960; there are current worrisome
outbreaks in Africa, Asia, and South America. Complications from the
Spanish flu killed approximately 20 million in a mere two years after its
outbreak in 1918. Smallpox, measles, typhus, and flu, which were introduced into the New World by the Spanish Conquistadores, killed 90% of
the native population. Entire Indian civilizations simply disappeared, and
the population dropped from 100 million to 10 million in just 150 years.

Bugs conquered the New World for Spain; they changed the course of history, just as HIV promises to do today. Still, it is most unlikely that AIDS will match these historic mortality figures.[3]

So what *is* the difference between "plague" and "epidemic"? Clearly, we do discriminate in our language. I would like to suggest that the discriminating criterion is subjective, not objective. Plague is a theological idea; it refers to an event that is imputed to God. In our emotional memory, plagues are terrifying, devastating, inescapable expressions of God's wrath and judgment. Those who die in them are targets, not victims; they are "Sinners in the Hands of an Angry God," to borrow Jonathan Edwards' eighteenth century sermon title. Epidemics, no matter how serious, pale into insignificance before direct manifestations of divine anger. The word "epidemic" is a term associated with the science of public health. Epidemics are understandable aspects of nature and manageable with modern skills. People who die in them are unfortunate victims, not sinners. Epidemics come from a nonjudgmental "Nature"; they arise from the lives of the people. Plagues come from God.[4]

The American media resurrected the fearsome label "plague" and applied it to AIDS. It is strange when you think of it. Our encounters with the Spanish flu of 1918, polio, and more recently Legionnaires' disease were never accorded that dread title. Why? The answer seems obvious. A just and compassionate God would never strike a Christian nation fighting barbarian Huns. He would never target children to suffer crippling paralysis and the embrace of an iron lung. Nor would He attack solid mainstream Americans meeting in patriotic convention. Thus those groups were visited by epidemics.

AIDS was an entirely different matter. In the epidemic's opening years in America, its main victims were male homosexuals living in New York City and San Francisco, "sinners" living in urban dens of iniquity. The Western biblical heritage linked with the American agrarian tradition to generate a powerful ideology of condemnation and avoidance.[5] The president of the Southern Baptist Association in 1986, clearly representing both traditions, proclaimed, "God created AIDS to show his displeasure into [sic] America's acceptance of the homosexual lifestyle." Baptist and Vatican orthodoxy met when Cardinal Kroll of Philadelphia pronounced the same judgment in 1987. Then American political orthodoxy spoke through Patrick Buchanan, President Reagan's Director of Media and Communication, who told us that "nature was finally exacting her price on homosexuals for having spilled their seed against her."[6] From the White House to millions of private houses, from thousands of pulpits, talk shows, news broadcasts, and editorials, AIDS was seen as God's punishment, a divine curse, and thus was labeled the "Gay Plague."[7]

Calling the AIDS epidemic a plague has the effect of indicting the ill, for in a plague the sick are not just sick, they are sinners. Illness itself is a mark of God's anger and is borne as a sign, a stigma, of that anger. The various signs, symptoms, or stigmata of affliction warn the righteous-well to shun the sick-sinner lest the contagion spread to them.[8] The plague mindset binds with tight theological knots the physical affliction and the putative moral failure. In Biblical and medieval times lepers were made to bear signs, wear bells, and live in quarantine leprosaria. During plague times the Pope authorized special ceremonies of penance to cleanse the spiritual atmosphere of the sin that God was presumably attacking; victims of the bubonic plague desperately tried to conceal their affliction to avoid condemnation.[9] Today proposals are heard to quarantine and even brand HIV infected individuals with some public mark of their physical and moral affliction, their crime against nature.

However, the only crime against nature is stupidity. People can and do get away with murder, but no person, no nation can escape the consequences of personal or public stupidity. A penalty is always assessed, and with little regard for constitutional notions of fair punishment. Early commentators on the epidemic ignored the fact that there is no such thing as a "gay" virus, one that targets people in terms of life style or sexual preference. They ignored the clear international evidence that HIV kills men, women, and children of all ages and attacks all races, nationalities, religions, and life styles. Their stupidity helped pave the way for the spread of the human immunode-ficiency virus, the deadliest and most "equal opportunity" enemy we have ever faced.

The harm done by this revival of the plague mentality is incalculable. What's in a word? Words can heal; words can kill. In the AIDS epidemic, "plague" is a lethal, killer word. The mindset expressed by the word excused the slowness and weakness of governmental action at the national, state, and local levels. Because of it, churches failed to provide the leadership that we rightfully expect of them—namely, compassionate understanding and vol-untary community care. I was amazed to read in the *San Francisco Chronicle* a headline stating, "Some churches *begin* counseling on AIDS" (my empha-sis). This in December 1987, four years after the problem was manifest in the Bay Area. In that same period, San Antonio's Northside Christian Church asked a long-standing, active member of the congregation "to voluntarily refrain from attending our gatherings" when it was discovered that he was suffering from AIDS. He died without the support of the church he had long supported. Two years later interfaith efforts to address the epidemic in a helpful and compassionate way were still hamstrung by the notable absence of Catholic and Southern Baptist leaders.[10] Can anyone who honors Christ truly believe that the man who raised the dead, fed the poor, embraced the outcast, and healed the sick would have approved? In times of crisis it becomes an obligation of the church and synagogue to lead, not run. Ignorance, fear, and the ancient doctrinal hatred of homosexuals flowed together to transform a deadly viral epidemic into an even deadlier "Gay Plague."

There was also a touch of wishful thinking on the part of mainstream Americans. After all, if AIDS was a judgment of God, then presumably the fate of the victims was deserved, and no extraordinary effort was called for to divert the calamity. President Reagan's budget officials resisted pressure to increase expenditures for AIDS-related programs, candidates in the 1984 elections totally ignored the developing crisis, and churches contented themselves with traditional moralizing. Average Americans went about their daily business, encouraged in the false belief that while AIDS was a sad affair, it was something that affected "them," not "us," and "they" (being undesirables anyway) were dispensable. In this heterosexual fantasy world, thinking about AIDS as a plague punishing homosexuals seemed to divert the Grim Reaper from most American front doors.[11]

Finally, in the darkest recess of the mind, in Dante's deepest level of Hell (reserved for leaders found unworthy of His mandate to rule justly), another and most ugly thought keeps breaking through the eternal lake of ice. With fervor and consistency, Americans have been taught that homosexuality is a perverse disposition, demonic or psychiatric in origin, to challenge nature and offend the Godly. If AIDS was commonly seen as divine retribution, then how many of our leaders believed that doing nothing was the appropriate response? What to do? Do nothing! Let God work His will; let the Reaper mow! For some, such an outcome might be seen as a way to help resolve the conundrums posed by homosexuality, drug abuse, and crime-ridden slums swarming with people of dubious pedigree and worth—an adaptation of Adolph Hitler's final solution.[12]

But then the children began to die. The nation was compelled to face a thorny problem of the plague mentality—the problem of the "innocent victim."[13] How does a reasonable person explain away the fact that God's aim seemed a trifle imprecise? Why would sexually innocent children, heterosexuals, women, hemophiliacs, health care workers, and others get caught in the fire and brimstone of divine retribution?

Cyprian, Bishop of Carthage, commenting on the Great Plague that was devastating his Mediterranean world of the third century A.D., gave the classic answer:

> Many of us are dying in this mortality, that is many of us are being freed from the world. This mortality is a bane to the Jews and pagans and enemies of Christ; to the servants of God it is a salutary departure. As to the fact that without any discrimination in the human race, the just are dying with the unjust, it is not for you to think that the destruction is a

common one for both the evil and the good. The just are called to refreshment, the unjust are carried off to torture; protection is more quickly given to the faithful, punishment to the faithless.[14]

Bishop Cyprian's position has a childlike simplicity. The rational mind cannot easily address it; it is a statement of faith. If you get sick and die, then it must be part of God's plan. Either you will be sent to Hell for your transgressions, or called to Heaven for your goodness. Since the human mind cannot know which will happen or why, it is best not to ask questions.

This explanation will hardly satisfy the modern mind. If we applied it consistently, then we should allow all who sicken from cholera, measles, flu, cancer, or the bubonic plague to die and be done with it. All these afflictions and more were at one time viewed as expressions of God's judgment. Nonetheless, echoes of Cyprian's position, usually presented as objective analysis, appear frequently in the press. For example, here is the commentary of nationally syndicated columnist John J. Kilpatrick:

> I would treat AIDS for what it is: a disease that mortally afflicts a tiny fraction of the population whose willful behavior results in the infection. The fellow who dies of sodomy is no more special than the fellow who dies of two packs of cigarettes a day.[15]

Kilpatrick's position has a superficial appeal. He states that "This disease overwhelmingly is a disease that afflicts two classes—drug addicts and homosexual men." Both contract the disease through voluntary, dangerous behavior and, consequently, there is no moral compulsion for society to exert itself unduly or feel much compassion.

Kilpatrick implies that his views are the result of objective analysis. Thus we can subject them to critical analysis. He is correct in stating that the spread of AIDS is partly traceable to the practice of sodomy, a word which today broadly denotes illegal oral or anal sex. There is little evidence that oral sex presents a major risk for the transmission of HIV; however, anal intercourse is another matter (see Chapter 5).[16] In the United States, anal intercourse has been a major mode of sexual expression within the homosexual and a secondary mode in the heterosexual community. Historically, anal intercourse has been a widespread technique of birth control, and today it is practiced, for example, in nations where for various reasons condoms are not readily available. There is absolutely no question that anal intercourse, without condom protection, is exceedingly dangerous in this age of AIDS. Kilpatrick is also correct in pointing to the use of unsterile needles among drug addicts as a significant path of transmission both here and in Europe. However, he is wrong to suggest that by eliminating these practices (or the people who practice them), the epidemic will be contained. It might be slowed; it will not be contained.

An enormous, frightening reservoir of possibly 10 million individuals around the globe are already infected. The overwhelming majority of these were not infected through the behavior that offends Kilpatrick.[17] Furthermore, most of the infected are unaware of the danger to themselves, or the danger they pose to others. These people undoubtedly will act as the source from which HIV can flow to the uninfected population. This is a fact of international life with AIDS. No one has formulated an acceptable policy to deal with it.

Another problem with the Kilpatrick analysis is the analogy drawn between smoking and lung cancer on the one hand, and sodomy and AIDS, on the other. He argues that both involve voluntary behaviors that, if stopped, would eliminate most of the problem. However, *the analogy is false*. AIDS is a communicable disease that can spread along many transmission routes; lung cancer is not. If all smoking stopped tomorrow, lung cancer would gradually become a rare ailment instead of the multibillion-dollar medical problem it is today. If all heterosexual and homosexual anal intercourse ceased tomorrow, and if all addicts began using sterile equipment, the human immunodeficiency virus would nonetheless continue its deadly way, multiplying and spreading. To be sure, its spread would be slowed, fewer people would be infected for a while, but the virus would remain undiminished in virulence.

Finally, we should never discount the capacity of HIV to mutate variants with more efficient modes of transmission. The evolution of *Yersinia pestis*, the agent of bubonic plague, should give us pause for thought in this regard. Over the course of its natural history, it evolved two transmission variants. First, there was the standard form by which disease was carried to the human host by fleas from infected rats, and which killed in from four hours (septicemic infection) to about three days (standard infection). Second, a pneumonic or airborne form, which could be conveyed from human to human through sneezes, coughs, and kissing, was fatal in about 12 hours. The private nightmare of many scientists working with the human immunodeficiency virus is that it will mutate the superbly efficient pneumonic form and become transmissible in the droplets of a sneeze, like a flu virus. There is absolutely no evidence, I repeat, *absolutely no evidence* that HIV has done so; on the other hand, there is absolutely no reason why it cannot. A genetic first cousin of HIV, the simian immunodeficiency virus (SIV) has evolved an as-yet rare variant that kills its monkey host in a mere six days, as compared with the many years it takes HIV to kill humans.[18] Three variants of our virus have already been isolated; these are HIV 1-oyi and HIV-2, both appearing in western rather than central Africa, and HIV-NDK which, if anything, seems even more virulent than HIV-1, which is the primary agent of the present epidemic.

Only at our peril dare we forget that the virus is a living entity. It will seek, like all living things, to ensure its survival by evolving biomolecular strategies to nullify, compensate for, or circumvent the drugs or behavioral changes we use to thwart it.[19] If HIV should mutate a pneumonic form before we have completed our basic research into the virus and developed some effective counter-measures, then every human being on this planet will be staring down the throat of a biologic black hole.

It is at this point that the true danger of such a view as Mr. Kilpatrick's becomes clear. If it prevails sufficiently to slow progress in research and treatment, we may all pay a dear price. However, notwithstanding its deficiencies and dangers, it is a position with great public appeal. This is not because of the facts or logic of it, but because it ties into our ancient Plague mindset. The key phrase in the editorial is, "a tiny fraction of the population." The fraction referred to is, of course, the "queers and junkies"—the undesirable and dispensable fraction of the population. Gallup polls show that about one-half of the adult population is sympathetic to this position, and I suspect the number is actually much higher. The poll results are undoubtedly affected by the fact that it is no longer considered good manners publicly to express one's prejudices. White prejudice against blacks, Gentile prejudice against Jews, and heterosexual prejudice against homosexuals are all deeply rooted in Western culture; it is unlikely that they have been eradicated, though they may be concealed by current forms of polite discourse.[20]

Kilpatrick reveals the real origins of his position by invoking the ancient category of the innocent victim. He advises us to take care of the kids and leave the rest of those sinners to God, a position that at the end of the decade emerged as one of the most influential views affecting the AIDS funding policy of the national and state governments. If by "innocent" victim he means to indicate those who did not by knowing, voluntary action bring the affliction upon themselves, then we must care as much for the homosexual and the drug user as for infected wives, infants, hemophiliacs, and heterosexuals. The truth of the matter is that most of those who are sick and dying now were infected as long as a decade ago, before anyone was aware of the existence, much less the danger of HIV.[21] No one can be said to have voluntarily exposed themselves to AIDS at that time; it was unknown. Even by the plague mentality's own terms, most of those currently ill are innocent victims.

The real mainspring of the plague position is revealed as old-fashioned hatred of homosexuals, a hatred that has been a festering boil on Western culture for millennia. This is supplemented by a disdain for those who use drugs other than those approved by the majority. For those with a more open and compassionate sensibility it should be evident that a plague is a church event, not unlike a heresy trial. A "plague" is not the work of God; it is a negative and self-destructive interpretation of the work of God. This interpretation has spread its poison into all aspects of our national response to the appearance of HIV in America.

One consequence of these stupidities has been that private and public funding for the care of those who are sick, except infants, has been hopelessly inadequate and slow to appear. The leadership of American society has simply dismissed the sick as dead, and "deservedly" so. Government money is overwhelmingly funnelled into research and, hopefully, preventive education. In Texas fully one-third of the State House of Representatives refused to sign a resolution offered in memory of the 3500 Texans who had died of AIDS and in appreciation of the private community groups that had provided the care that the state had withheld. The same legislature also severely cut state grant funds supporting hospice and home daycare, for fear the money might fall into the hands of homosexual caregivers;[22] the result has been to force AIDS patients into the much more expensive, and less appropriate, hospital environment or to deny terminal care altogether.[23] There is no question that our cultural prejudices, our homophobia in particular, have contributed to a slow and stupid response to the epidemic, a response that can be measured in deaths—a sad commentary upon a people who profess to honor Christ.[24]

Clearly, America desperately needs presidential leadership in order to effectively address the HIV epidemic. Only the White House pulpit has the power to neutralize the plague pulpits and give us the confidence to assay, fund, and fight the battle against AIDS. Given the strength of our cultural bigotries, the President must constantly remind the nation that it faces a public health emergency, an epidemic, not a religious crisis. The only moral dimension involved in this epidemic relates to the adequacy and compassion of our national response. For reasons time will sort out, President Ronald Reagan was unwilling to exert this kind of leadership; Congress forced his reluctant administration to develop the programs of the early years. Someone must have asked him, or perhaps he asked himself, "What should I do?" History records the answer: "Do nothing."

President George Bush is offered the challenge and opportunity to set an appropriate national tone, and build a constructive government agenda to confront HIV. At a conference of the National Leadership Coalition on AIDS in March 1990, he did call for compassionate and nondiscriminatory care for the sick but stopped short of concrete proposals. It is a step, but just a step, in the right direction.[25] As the National Commission on AIDS pointed out, rhetoric must be matched with funded programs.[26] Even while the President spoke, the funds available from both private foundations and his administration to meet the various costs of providing care were, in fact, diminishing.[27]

Properly considered, I am not talking about presidential inclinations preferences, or policy choices, but rather the most important of presidential responsibilities. Decisions on the budget, the make-up of the weapons system, the funding of Medicare, and the like can be made and are made by many competent people in authority. However, only the President of the United States, who is our head of state, can lead the entire nation down constructive paths. We distinguish our great leaders from the merely competent ones by their willingness to educate the public in attitudes and policies that, in the long term, will benefit the commonwealth—not Republicans or Democrats, but the whole people. George Washington set the precedent for this overriding presidential responsibility in his "Farewell Address to the Nation," and we have measured our leaders by their success in building upon this foundation. President Roosevelt, in his "Quarantine Speech" of 1937, warned Americans that, whether they liked it or not, they could not isolate themselves from the affairs of the world. It was an unpopular message, one that a large segment of the nation did not want to hear. By leading the way, he inspired a massive public educational effort, joined by ministers, journalists, educators, and all ranks of public officials, to wean the public away from its foolish and self-destructive isolationist position. He began preparing the public mind for the events that would tragically unfold in the Japanese bombardment of Pearl Harbor. After the battlefield conclusion of World War II, Winston Churchill set the tone for Western public attitudes toward Stalin's Soviet Union with his famous "Iron Curtain" speech. John Kennedy, in his inaugural and "Berlin Wall" addresses, defined fundamental American domestic and international positions in an increasingly dangerous world—a world that held its breath during the Cuban missile crisis. Now it is George Bush's turn to lead the way; his opportunity to move beyond competence to greatness.

Of course, the deadly virus will not be contained by words alone, even healing presidential words. People, facilities, and money must all be mobilized and targeted, and we all must do what we can to create and administer enlightened national, state, and local policy. But as the chairman of Levi Strauss & Co. so rightly observed, our best efforts will be of little avail "if there is darkness in the White House."[28] President Bush must do the job that only a president can do; he must help the nation see "Demon Plague" for what he is, a dangerous theological throwback to our past, that serves only to confuse and frustrate the present.

Notes

1. Professor William H. McNeill, an eminent historian at the University of Chicago, is the author of many noted books, among which is *Plagues and Peoples* (New York: Anchor, 1976), p. 289. At the point of my quotation from Prof. McNeill's book, he refers to Richard Fiennes, *Man, Nature and Disease* (London, 1964), p. 124, which projects possible population dieoffs in case of the spread of new agents.
2. S. I. Hayakawa, *Language in Action* (New York: Harcourt, Brace & Co., 1941).
3. McNeill, *Plagues and Peoples*, Chap. 5.
4. Consider the structure of the word *epidemic*. *Epi*, from, prefixed to *demos*, people. An epidemic is of and from the people.
5. An ideological tradition deeply imbedded in the American mind, which goes back through Jefferson to Rousseau, asserts that virtue resides in the plain country folk who make their living by honestly tilling the good earth. The city is viewed with suspicion as a place of corruption, venality, and sin. In the fight over repeal of prohibition in Oklahoma, for example, the "dry" ministers warned their parishioners that Oklahoma would become "like New York City" if prohibition were repealed. See Robert S. Walker and Samuel C. Patterson, *Oklahoma Goes Wet: The Repeal of Prohibition in Oklahoma* (Eagleton Institute, Cases in Practical Politics, Rutgers, The State University, New York: McGraw-Hill, 1960).
6. Paul Monette, *Borrowed Time: An AIDS Memoir* (New York: Harcourt, Brace, Jovanovich, 1988).
7. The English experience was remarkably parallel to the American. Peter Aggleton and Hilary Thomas, *Social Aspects of AIDS* (London: Falmer Press, 1988).
8. Susan Sontag, *AIDS and Its Metaphors* (New York: Farrar, Straus & Giroux, 1988).
9. The old nursery rhyme we all learned as children:

> Ring around the rosy,
> Pockets full of posies
> Ashes, ashes,
> All fall down.

is a grim expression of this. "Ring around the rosy" refers to the physical appearance of the pustules that erupted on the skin of the infected. "Posies" were the aromatic herbs the infected carried in an attempt to disguise the sick smell emitted by the boils. "Ashes" refers to the practice of burning clothing, bedding, and sometimes the victim. Finally, "All fall down"—in the end, death conquered.
10. "Religious Leaders Exhorted to Press U.S. on AIDS Crisis," *New York Times*, December 5, 1989, p. A14. A report on a large interfaith meeting in Atlanta at the Carter Presidential Center.
11. The fundamentalist American Council of Christian Churches, which claims to speak for 2 million people, asserts the plague mentality forcefully and without qualification. However, many churches find themselves caught between the pull of classic plague doctrine and a more contemporary view. The bishops of the Catholic Church, meeting at their national conference in Baltimore, November 1989, issued ambiguous statements reflecting the apprehension that, if they flatly denied divine authorship of the epidemic they might thereby open the door to

more basic questions as to God's intervention in mundane affairs. Doctrinal conservatives of all faiths generally shied away from any statement that could be construed as a departure from the traditional position of homosexuality as sin, even if it produced the logical, if questionably Christian result that they approved the epidemic as an instance of divine retribution. After all, how can one *not* approve of divine action of any kind? Heresy lurks in such questioning. Various polls indicate that at least 25% of the population will admit to the "divine retribution" view. See the New York Times Service report, which appeared in various newspapers on November 19, 1989, relating some of these conflicts of conscience. Also see J. Gordon Melton, *The Churches Speak on AIDS* (Santa Barbara, CA: Institute for the Study of American Religion, 1989). Melton is the director of the Institute.

12. For those whose first reaction to this conjecture is to dismiss it out of hand, I would suggest several works: James H. Jones, *Bad Blood: The Tuskegee Syphilis Experiment* (New York: Free Press, 1981), pp. 17–48. Jones examines the theories of racial inferiority that were used to justify the use of blacks in syphilis medical experimentation. For example, nineteenth century white physicians explained the high rate of syphilis in the black population on the ground that blacks were immoral and promiscuous (exactly the perception of gays today). Black vice, in turn, reflected the fact that "personal restraints on self-indulgence did not exist because the smaller brain of the Negro had failed to develop a center for inhibiting sexual behavior." On the AIDS epidemic as seen by one of the most important gay activists in the nation, see Larry Kramer, *Reports from the Holocaust: The Making of an AIDS Activist* (New York: St. Martin's Press, 1989). And finally, Evelynn Hammond's provocative article, "Race, Sex, AIDS, the Construction of 'Other'," *Radical America* 20, no. 6 (Nov./Dec. 1986): 28–38.

13. For example, the story of little Celeste Garrian, who died at the age of 12 in 1989, after having been born with AIDS in 1977, and suffering the affliction her entire life. She survived longer than any other child born with AIDS. Bruce Lambert, *New York Times*, November 7, 1989, p. 1.

14. Cyprian, *De Mortalitate* (Hannon, transl.), as quoted in McNeill, *Plagues and Peoples*, p. 122.

15. *San Antonio Express-News*, June 1988.

16. See Chapter 5.

17. Dieter Koch Weser and Hannelore Vanderschmidt (eds.), *The Heterosexual Transmission of AIDS in Africa* (Cambridge, MA: ABT Books, 1988).

18. "Fast-Killing AIDS in Monkeys," *New York Times*, June 14, 1990, p. A12.

19. A most disturbing development is the resurgence of old diseases, like syphilis and measles, in new resistant forms. Brian Goldman, "'Old' Diseases Stage a Comeback—And Its Not Child's Play This Time," *Observer* (American College of Physicians) 9, no. 10 (November 1989): 1.

20. R. J. Blendon, et al. (Harvard AIDS Institute, Harvard School of Public Health) "Discrimination Against People with AIDS: A Public's Perspective," *New England Journal of Medicine* 319 (October 13, 1988): 1022–1026. A. Comfort, "AIDS: Public Panic," *Journal of the Royal Society of Medicine* 81, no. 10 (October 1988): 618. This destructive mentality is clearly fostered in the nation's influential evangelical ministry. TV preachers like Jimmy Swaggart, Oral Roberts, Jerry Falwell, and Pat Robertson earnestly preach the plague mindset, and their followers dutifully reflect their position. See the August 31, 1987

Gallup Report on public attitudes toward AIDS sufferers, which pinpoints "evangelicals and those who have not completed high school as the groups most likely to see AIDS as a punishment from God."

21. D. Huminer and J. B. Rosenfeld, "AIDS in the Pre-AIDS Era," *Review of Infectious Diseases* 9 (1987): 1102–1108.

22. As an example, the Texas Department of Health refused to renew the funding for the Dallas AIDS Resource Center's free food bank because the center is operated by the Dallas Gay Alliance. *Austin American-Statesman*, January 4, 1990, p. A1.

23. *San Antonio Express-News*, Kay Northcott's comment, "AIDS Bill Emphasizes Criminality," May 19, 1989.

24. John David Dupree, Ph.D., Glen Margo, MSW, "Homophobia, AIDS and the Health Care Professional," in *FOCUS: A Guide to AIDS Research* (San Francisco, CA: The AIDS Health Project of the University of California San Francisco, 1988).

25. *New York Times*, March 30, 1990, p. A1. The membership of the National Leadership Coalition on AIDS consists of the executives of large businesses.

26. See the *Report of the National AIDS Commission*, December 1989, which challenges the President to "match rhetoric with action."

27. Marisa Venegas and Tom Watkins, "AIDS Funders of Last Resort Cutting Community Services," *Medical Tribune, International Medical News Weekly*, January 11, 1990, p. 1. "AIDS Groups Are Worried by Looming Fiscal Crisis," *New York Times*, May 6, 1990, p. 19.

28. *New York Times*, March 30, 1990, p. A1. Remarks of Robert D. Haas, chairman of Levi Strauss & Co., at meeting, March 29, 1990, sponsored by the National Leadership Coalition on AIDS.

2

==

Parasites and People: Cohabitors of Earth

THE HUMAN IMMUNODEFICIENCY VIRUS

Webster's Collegiate Dictionary defines a parasite as "a plant or animal living in, on, or with, some other living organism at whose expense it obtains food, shelter, or the like." We all "live in, off, or with" some other organism—the parent and child relationship, for example. The key element of the definition is the phrase "at whose expense." There is the sense that parasites somehow take without giving, and that the relationship between host and parasite is unilateral and destructive. If the parasite has made any positive contribution it must be on the very broad level of evolutionary development. Parasites come in all shapes and sizes—mistletoe, ticks, mosquitoes, *Y. pestis*, and our own HIV-1, 2.[1] The character of parasitism also varies. Some use the host for support and shelter, others for food, others for some phase of their life cycle, while for still others the host is their total environment. HIV is a retroviral intracellular microparasite that spends its entire life cycle in the bloodstream of the human host. Its classification as a parasite stems from the fact that it uses its genetic template to convert the cellular activity of key human cells into a process that replicates the viral cells. In effect, it is able to convert our cells into surrogate mothers giving birth to an ever increasing quantity of HIV cells. It is worth emphasizing that our virus is *our* virus, it is the *human* immunodeficiency virus. Even its genetic structure overlaps ours.[2] HIV does not naturally occur in any other animal.

When it came to the notice of the Western world it inspired the usual cold war, conspiracy, and extraterrestrial theories of origin. Soviet agents spread rumors in Africa that it was a genetically engineered product of American biological warfare spread by the CIA. More imaginatively, it was suggested

14

that HIV made its earthly debut riding on a comet from outerspace.[3] HIV's biologic origin may never be known with certainty, but it probably appeared as a human pathogen sometime in the last 100 years.[4] In 1987 Dr. Robert C. Gallo of the National Cancer Institute suggested that it might have been a mutation, several times removed, of a similar virus infecting the African green monkey, *Ceropithecus aethiops*, which may have cross-infected a human at some time. The green monkey is hunted for food in Central Africa, so a cross-infection seemed possible. Research following up Gallo's suggestion indicated that the etiology of HIV was more complex. While HIV and SIV (simian immunodeficiency virus) did have much in common, advancing research made it seem more likely that SIV was a mutation of the human virus HIV-2 rather than the other way around.[5]

The beginning point for understanding the cataclysm we call an epidemic is the concession that from the standpoint of the natural world it is not a cataclysm at all. It is just another event like an earthquake, a volcanic eruption, or the birth or death of a star or a species. Writers have awarded our species many designations, most of them complimentary (man the toolmaker, the risen ape, and so on), conceding pride of place only to God. Whatever else we are, it is clear that we are the most egotistical species. Because we generally believe that the universe revolves around us, we often forget that the first law of organic nature is that there is no such thing as a free lunch. Even though we are evolution's most successful, top-of-the-line predator, still, we cannot eat without being eaten.

Masters of all we survey, we tend to ignore what we cannot see, a humble, infinitesimally small virus quite capable of destroying us in the process of reproducing itself. The virus stands at the beginning step of life while we stand at the complex end of it; it is humbling, or should be. We are in the initial stages of a world epidemic that has the potential of reversing past trends of global population growth.[6] Balanced perspective begins with understanding that this epidemic is a natural event, with the concession that HIV is part of nature just as we are, that it has a role in the unimaginably intricate chain of being just as we do, and that it is very unlikely that either of us will eradicate the other. Our problem is to find a way of living with the virus, instead of dying from it.

A good place to start is to see HIV as just one among many organisms that live in, on, or with us. The illustrative list in Table 2.1 is meant merely to display some of the popularly known microbes with a taste for you and me, and to place HIV in company with its companions. Table 2.1 contains some of the common assaults upon our species. It ignores many rare but deadly ones such as the viral hemorrhagic fevers, or widespread debilitating ones like schistosomiasis, endemic in the fresh water of many nations. The point

TABLE 2.1   Human Diseases

VIRAL DISEASES		BACTERIAL DISEASES	
DISEASE	USUAL MODE OF TRANSMISSION	DISEASE	USUAL MODE OF TRANSMISSION
Smallpox	Airborne	Pneumonias	Airborne
Measles	Airborne	Diphtheria	Airborne
Influenzas	Airborne	Tuberculoses	Airborne
Mononucleosis	Oral contact	Lyme disease	Ticks
Enteroviruses (65 types)	Stool/hand/mouth	*Salmonella*	Stool/hand/food
Hepatitis B NonA/nonB	Stool/hand/mouth Transfusion	Leprosy	Prolonged close contact
Warts	Skin to skin	*Staphylococci*	Open wounds
Arboviruses	Mosquitoes, ticks	Bubonic plague	Fleas, airborne
Herpes simplex	Sexual contact	Gonorrhoea	Sexual contact
Cytomegalovirus	Sexual contact	Syphilis	Sexual contact
HIV-associated diseases (including AIDS)	**Sexual contact, *in utero*, trans- fusion**	Cholera and typhus	Contaminated water

to be emphasized is that we are the preferred environment for a long list of bugs. Like it or not, we are part of the chain of existence. HIV is dramatically reminding us of that fact of life.

While it is not unique in targeting a human host, HIV is certainly the most dangerous and insidious viral enemy we have ever faced.[7] Prior to 1981 it was just a suspicion, an apprehension that there was "something out there." Physicians and epidemiologists in Africa, Europe, and America were recording a puzzling new collection of ailments that defied classification and resisted all medical interventions. In 1981 five cases of *Pneumocystis carinii* pneumonia (PCP) and 26 cases of Kaposi's sarcoma (KS) were reported to the Centers for Disease Control (CDC); both afflictions were medically known, but rare. All cases were in homosexual men from New York and California. In 1982 the CDC officially classified the new collection of clinical conditions as a syndrome, and began monitoring a now officially recognized illness. Later a separate classification was established for children. The first cases of hemophiliac and transfusion infections were also recorded in 1982. Still, no one knew what was causing the newly observed health problems and deaths. Then in 1983 Luc Montagnier, leading a team of scientists at France's Pasteur Institute, isolated HIV. The French discovery was supported by findings from America's National Cancer Institute.[8] Finally, in 1983 the first cases of heterosexual male-to-female transmission were recorded. By this time HIV, spreading quietly for at least 30 years, had infected as many as 10 million people worldwide, and at least 1 million Americans.[9]

HIV is an approximately round, very complex retrovirus of about 100 nanoMicrons in diameter (one ten-thousandth of a millimeter), whose envelope or surface membrane has molecular spikes (glycoproteins 120 and 41) that enable it to attach to and fuse with human cells having CD4 molecular receptors on their envelope surface (Fig. 2.1).[10] HIV's membrane surrounds a dense inner core containing various protein molecules, enzymes, and amino acids. When the virus encounters a cell with CD4 receptors, it attaches itself and disgorges its genetic materials into the host cell. It is at its most destructive to us when it attaches to and uses the T helper/inducer lymphocyte cells—commonly called T4 cells. The proper functioning of T4s is essential to an effective antibody response to disease pathogens—from common colds to pneumonia—entering our bodies. Upon infecting a T4 cell, HIV commences a process that replicates the virus while eventually destroying the host cell. Over a period of time this so seriously compromises the immune system that survival itself is threatened. AIDS is our first experience with a viral-based primary immune-regulating illness. HIV's life cycle directly assaults the very walls that nature has constructed over the eons of hominid evolution to protect us against bacterial and viral invaders like HIV.

The virus is sensitive to its environment. It thrives and is exceedingly tough in its natural environment, but is fragile outside of it. Fortunately a wide range of common materials like household detergents, bleach, alcohol, iodine, hydrogen peroxide, and even human saliva are toxic to it.[11] A good deal of public misunderstanding relating to the probabilities of transmission and the possibilities of developing a vaccine stem from the virus's dual tough but fragile character.[12]

HIV has a family and a life cycle. It is part of the lentivirus branch of a larger family group known as retroviruses; the prefix *lenti* expresses the fact that members of this branch produce an infection that develops very slowly—in the case of HIV, over many years. It is one of about 14 genetically related microbes that trace their ancestry back over millions of

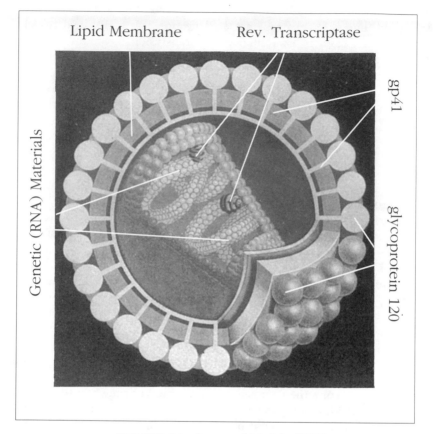

FIGURE 2.1   Structural Model of HIV

Source: José Esparza, "Prospects for a Vaccine," *World Health: The Magazine of the World Health Organization*, October 1989, p. 10.

years, perhaps to some common origin. Currently two very close cousins of HIV are known, both of which are deadly, although neither is as widespread.[13] All members of the lentivirus family seem to have one common characteristic—they make whatever animal they inhabit very sick, whether it be cattle, horses, sheep, chickens, reptiles, mice, monkeys, or your pet cat. Many of them produce in animal hosts effects similar to those that HIV produces in us. We are not alone.

HIV's Life Cycle and the Tactics of Combat

Since its discovery in 1983, retrovirologists have traced the stages of HIV's life cycle in considerable detail. It is important to have some general understanding of the process, because it is on the foundation of this knowledge that our strategies of cure or treatment must rest. The technical language describing it is the arcane language of molecular biology; understanding that what follows is a gross oversimplification, allow me to cast the process as occurring in four stages and in terms of familiar images (see Fig. 2.2).[14]

Stage 1, Injection: Imagine that HIV is a small boat of guerrilla raiders launched, sometimes by you, sometimes by others, into the river of your bloodstream. HIV circulates in the currents of the bloodstream until it encounters a likely docking site. It can only dock at wharves the configuration of which match that of the boat. Various cell-wharves offer such facilities.[15] Stage 2, Infection: When the virus boat docks at the T4 wharf, the raiders take over and unload their cargo of replication materials. Stage 3, Replication: The patrol leader (an enzyme called *reverse transcriptase*) directs T4's residents in building and stocking new boats for further raiding. Stage 4, Recapitulation: Finally, they launch the new, freshly provisioned boats into your bloodstream to start the process over again, but this time in greater numbers. As parting thanks to the T4 facility, they frequently destroy it.[16] Within the framework of these four stages it is possible to gain some appreciation for the incredible complexity of fighting HIV.

INJECTION

The first stage, of course, involves the introduction of the virus into the bloodstream. Technically it is not a stage of infection, but the necessary prelude to infection. If the virus never enters a human cell, even though it is within the bloodstream, then no infection takes place. This may seem an empty distinction, but it is critical in Stage 2, as we shall see. Injection of the virus into the bloodstream can occur as a result of carelessness in the handling of infected materials, just plain rotten luck as in a hospital accident, or culpable industrial negligence in transfusion of blood or blood products. It can also result from another kind of transfusion, as when contaminated syringes or needles are used by intravenous (IV) drug users. It can result from being born to infected parents. Finally, HIV injection can result from unprotected (condomless) sex with an infected partner, male or female. Various other means of transmission have been suggested (kissing, insect bites, and toilet seats, for example). However, responsible research now resting upon literally hundreds of thousands of cases has failed to document

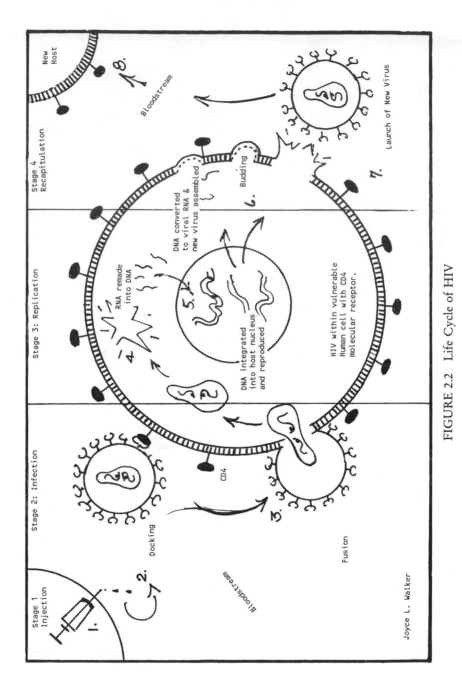

FIGURE 2.2 Life Cycle of HIV

these other routes. They are within the realm of theoretic possibility (see Chapter 5), but not life's real probabilities.[17]

These various routes require different strategies to prevent initial injection. Minimization of blood transference in accident and health care situations can only be achieved through ongoing educational campaigns within the industry, and the provision of as much operational safety as is consistent with the job. Measures can range from hospital training seminars for paramedics, through the development of new protective materials, to rules requiring double-gloving in surgery. The health care industry is now acutely aware of the dangers, and new protocols and training programs are developing rapidly.[18] The general efficacy of protective procedures designed for health care workers is attested by the very small number worldwide who have been infected in the line of duty.[19] However, extra protection does not come free. Estimates in late 1990 put the additional health care costs at $337 million/year.[20]

Dr. Marcus Conant, a physician at the University of California, San Francisco School of Medicine, has published the recommendation that a physician suffering a needle stick injury immediately commence a self-prescribed AZT regimen as a way of decreasing risk of seroconversion.[21] However, no measures can eliminate risk; some is inevitable, and the possibilities are definitely not negligible. It is estimated that one in every 250 accidental needle-sticks sustained by health workers caring for seropositive patients results in viral transmission and, further, that a surgeon 10% of whose patients are HIV+ has a 1:200 chance of becoming infected during the course of each working year.[22]

Attention to the possibility of injection during health care procedures has tended to focus on the problem of the health care worker, but there are many more instances of patients being infected in what can only be called health care industry negligence. One of the most tragic cases developed in the Soviet Union in the period from 1981 through 1989. As reported at Montreal's International Conference on AIDS, a Russian male working in Guinea was infected and then infected his wife upon returning to the Soviet Union. She became pregnant; the baby was born infected in 1984. The child sickened and was hospitalized in Elista, capital of the Kalmuk Republic on the Caspian Sea. The hospital was operating with an inadequate supply of hypodermic syringes due to a national shortage.[23] The nurses, departing from proper procedure, used the same needle for multiple patient injections, and the original infection spread to 51 other children in the pediatric ward. Then one of the newly infected infants was transferred to a hospital in Volgorod where exactly the same thing happened, spreading the infection to 22 more. In addition, 8 mothers were infected, possibly through breastfeeding—their babies' mouths had bleeding sores and they were infected through minute cracks in their nipples. All told, 81 infections can be traced back to the original Guinea contact, 78 of them attributable to health care negligence.[24] A popular Soviet weekly, *Ogonyok*, prophesied that unless the scarcity of antiseptic hospital conditions is corrected, AIDS could spread to millions of Soviets by the year 2000.[25]

By far the largest number of individuals infected through industrial negligence were infected in the United States as a result of the transfusion of contaminated blood and blood products. The story of the mulish reluctance of America's blood bank managers to begin screening procedures is one of the saddest chapters in the history of our early nonresponse to the threat of AIDS. As early as 1982 experts, studying patterns of infection in hemophiliac recipients of blood products, considered it highly probable that HIV could be transmitted by blood transfusion.[26] In late 1982 and early 1983 President Reagan's Food and Drug Administration (the agency charged with regulating the blood bank industry) issued recommendations to reduce the risk of possible transmission. In 1983–1984 the virus was isolated, but not until 1985 did the FDA issue mandatory screening regulations.

The position of industry leaders was that no one had "proved conclusively" that AIDS could be transmitted through transfusion. Lacking such evidence, screening was too expensive. The industry position reminds one of the tobacco industry's persistent claim that "100% certain" scientific proof of a causal link between smoking and lung cancer has not been established. By the time blood bank administrators bowed to the mounting evidence and implemented the FDA regulations, many thousands of hemophiliacs and approximately 12,000 surgical patients were added to the growing list of AIDS victims.[27] The Ryan White Comprehensive AIDS Act of 1990 (see Chapter 6) requires the states to develop public information campaigns targeting people who received transfusions between January 1, 1978 and April 1, 1985, and inform them of the availability and need for health services.[28] There are now 200 to 300 lawsuits pending against various blood banks for contaminated transfusions.[29]

The problem of contaminated blood has been reasonably well addressed by now. The supply has never been and will never be 100% free of possible disease contaminants, for nothing is absolutely safe. But probably it is as good as one can get anywhere in the world today.[30] However, I would not want to receive a transfusion in Mexico, Central or South America, the Caribbean, Africa, the Middle East, the Eastern Mediterranean, India, or Southeast Asia—a fair chunk of the world. U.S. government operations with contingents in these areas (such as the U.S. military, the Peace Corps, the State Department, the Central Intelligence Agency) fly their personnel to Europe or America or use previously banked blood when transfusions are needed. It is not a question of the nations involved being unwilling to screen;

it is usually that they are unable to screen for economic or technological reasons.[31]

America is not without its own problems. The cases of Dr. David J. Acer, dentist, and Dr. Rudolph Almaraz, surgeon, both of whom reportedly died of AIDS, promise to radically change the prevailing rules regarding practice and notification. The position of the health care profession prior to 1991 was that the patient had no need and no right to know the HIV status of health care workers assigned to his or her case. However, it may be that Dr. Acer infected some of his patients. And in Dr. Almaraz's case, his employer (Sloan-Kettering Cancer Center) has offered HIV tests to about 1800 patients to ascertain whether the infection had been passed on. It is probable that the risk of doctor-to-patient transmission is low. However, given that the entire purpose of medical intervention is to improve the health of the patient, it seems clear that no avoidable adverse condition—be it a septic condition of the surgery or the health of workers—can be permitted. The Centers for Disease Control have reports of 40 surgeons, 588 nonsurgical physicians, 144 dental workers, and 1063 nurses who have been diagnosed with AIDS. How many HIV+ health care professionals are currently practicing no one knows. The Acer, Almaraz, and other cases persuaded the American Medical and American Dental Associations to issue new guidelines in January 1991 stating that health care workers had an ethical obligation to inform patients of a seropositive status. It remains to be seen whether state health departments will accept and enforce these new guidelines.[32]

There are also instances of what can only be called accident-accidents—events of so unpredictable and bizarre a character that there is little or no conceivable protection. I have in mind, for example, the case of an American tourist in Rwanda who was seriously injured along with other passengers in a bus crash. His open wounds were splattered with the blood of other passengers piled on top of him; one of them was HIV+, and the infection was transmitted.[33] Millions of Americans travel each year in Third World countries where the conditions of life in all respects are more hazardous, where HIV prevalence is higher, where the male-female seroprevalence ratio is close to even, and where medical facilities themselves may be a significant source of infection.

Then there are the children infected in the womb, in the very citadel of life itself, in the birthing process, or through breastfeeding. A child born to an infected mother has about a 25% chance of infection. Eighty-one percent of the pediatric cases in the United States can be linked to IV drug use.[34] The Centers for Disease Control project that we will have between 10,000 and 20,000 cases of pediatric AIDS by 1991. The World Health Organization estimates that by the year 2000, the number of HIV+ children in sub-Saharan Africa will number in the millions.

In America most AIDS babies will be born in a hospital, and most will never leave it. It is sobering to realize that an entire group of infants will come into and go out of our world without experiencing the holding, the bonding, and the love that forges a human being from the raw material of our species. Statistical analyses indicate that about 20% of infected newborns will develop AIDS within the first year of life and die during the next; the rest will progress to AIDS at the rate of 8% per year.[35] A quick tour of an AIDS pediatric ward would probably stifle most of the moralistic posturing about God's wrath. The tour would also illustrate a facet of our response to the epidemic. The national government and various charitable groups are funding pediatric care lavishly (it is politically acceptable to help the innocent victims), but adult care parsimoniously. Unfortunately, good support does not change the result. Children are born to drunken parents, cruel and sadistic parents, careless and improvident parents, and parents who abandon them. Most of them survive it all. None survive AIDS.[36]

Finally, there is transmission as a result of our own high-risk behavior, risky sex, or injecting drugs with contaminated syringes (the Soviet and Romanian pediatric tragedies are instructive here). Prior to 1985 no one could be held accountable for failing to avoid behaviors that were and are risky in terms of AIDS for the simple reason that there was too little information, too much confusion, and no truly authoritative guidance. But nature does not require culpability or intentionality in any sense. It is enough that you do something that, in fact, is dangerous; you pay—no if's, and's, or but's. Most of those who are sick and dying currently are in this group. They were infected in the late 1970s or early 1980s before anyone was really informed as to the nature of the illness, its forms of transmission, or the possible scope of the epidemic.

Increasingly from 1985 to the present, the possibility of being honestly ignorant is very slowly decreasing as government agencies, churches, and educational institutions gradually educate the public. At this moment, about the only weapons we have to fight this epidemic are educational campaigns such as that mounted by former U.S. Surgeon General Koop at the national level, local efforts sponsored by America's thousands of AIDS service organizations, and an increasing number of educational programs sponsored by schools, businesses, and churches. In aggregate, they are simultaneously impressive and inadequate. We are rapidly learning how little we know about how to convince people to change their basic ways or, indeed, even how to reach them with a message they can assimilate. I have been involved in local phases of this national educational effort and have been humbled by the discovery that I knew much less about teaching than I thought; the elaborate plans—posters, pamphlets, programs—always sound great to the middle-class, educated warriors around the conference table, but absolutely bomb when put into effect. Still, people are learning and, in any event, they are all we have. Anyone who, for reasons of sexual prudishness, religious commitment, homophobic sexual prejudice, or antipathy to drug use impedes these efforts is, very simply, an ally of the epidemic.

INFECTION

If by one means or the other, the virus is injected into the human bloodstream, then conditions are set for stage 2; the boat is launched. An entirely different set of problems arises and the newly seropositive person has fundamentally lost control over the ultimate health of his or her body. There is nothing that the individual can now do other than live in such a way as to enhance general health, avoid contracting or transmitting further sexually transmitted diseases (STDs), and follow treatment protocols. Upon infection, at least for the person infected, the public health campaigns of stage 1 have failed. Now matters are in the hands of research and clinical medicine. What can be done?

The virus will encounter a human cell that it chemically recognizes as a potential host, and "dock." Technically, docking involves the attachment of HIV's surface coat molecule gp120 to the CD4 molecule found on the surface of a number of human cells. Docking is followed by a fusion of HIV with the host cell through the action of another HIV surface molecule, gp41.[37] The vulnerable cells of our immune system are the T4, the T8, and the B lymphocytes, as well as the monocytes/macrophages. In addition, the virus can invade the glial cells of the brain and central nervous system.

HIV adversely affects in some way the function of any cell it enters, but by far its most significant damage is through its disruption of the T4 cell.[38] This cell is the master organizer and dispatcher of the immune system's response to attackers which, like HIV, integrate themselves into our various cells. In what is known as "cell-mediated" response, T4 directs the production of antibodies and mobilizes them against the foreign, "non-self" biological presence. When HIV fuses to a T4 cell, fatal human infection commences.

There are two major strategies: (1) to prevent the docking and fusion of HIV to a host cell, or (2) to enhance the body's ability to destroy free virus or virus-infected cells. The first approach involves interfering with the process of docking so that the virus is left to drift, eventually to be destroyed by immune system defenders or by a specially targeted toxin.[39] There are many different drugs being tested to frustrate the process of docking and penetration. AL-721 (active lipid 721) attempts to alter the organization of the HIV membrane (to make it more "slippery," in layman's terms) so that it will be unable to bind to the CD4 receptor. AL-721 has been a favorite "underground" or home remedy because it is easily made from available materials, but its effectiveness has yet to be established. Another approach has been to load the blood system with decoys in the form of recombinant soluble CD4 to which HIV could attach harmlessly. Still other approaches seek to attach additional molecules to the CD4 receptor. The wharf is thus structurally altered so that the boat will not fit, and the HIV gp120 will be unable to attach.[40]

The second strategy involves enhancing the body's natural immune response, as is done with the polio vaccine, so that the invading virus is overwhelmed. This involves the complicated business of producing a vaccine that will create a cellular "memory" of HIV before an individual is infected. Then, if and when the person is invaded by HIV, the body's immune system will be able to mount an immediate and decisive defense.

The search for agents that will meet the needs of one or the other strategy is furious and many faceted but so far without the kind of result we all want.[41] Most of the progress has been on drugs that slow or partially impede HIV's progress without stopping it altogether. As far as a preventive vaccine is concerned, there is little expectation of one in this century. Dr. Jonas Salk announced, in June 1989, that his research team had made some advances in producing a postinfection vaccine, that is, a treatment or therapeutic vaccine designed to stimulate the body's own defense mechanisms and thus significantly slow the progression to AIDS. This was followed by the successful formulation of a preinfection simian AIDS vaccine in December 1989.[42]

These encouraging announcements, as well as research presented at the Sixth International Conference on AIDS in June 1990, indicate that vaccines are possible. However, speculation about the possibilities of a vaccine must be understood in the context of the overall difficulties involved. One of the principals of the simian virus research team cautioned that "The day when we come up with a human vaccine against AIDS is still far off."[43] The scientific mood remains cautious. One noted virologist stated, "The development of a [preventive] vaccine against AIDS is hindered by the worst possible confluence of viral and pathogenic factors that seem to preclude any simple or easy resolution in the foreseeable future."[44] The press releases of the U.S. Surgeon General, the National Institutes of Health, and various other groups have uniformly emphasized the difficulties and improbability of a human vaccine in less than a decade of research and testing.[45]

There are all sorts of problems that impede vaccine development.[46] One of the more ironic is that a vaccine that stimulates the production of necessary cells to defeat HIV might actually stimulate the production of more HIV. Since HIV integrates its genetic material into the host cell's material, any division of the host cell in response to the injection (vaccination) of a foreign substance automatically creates new viral materials. Seen from HIV's standpoint it is a brilliant strategy; seen from ours, it is a deadly and macabre minuet. Another major problem derives from the hypermutability and variability of HIV. It is customary, especially in general literature such as this work, to speak of the HIV as though it were just one virus. Actually, it seems to be a complex family of rapidly mutating viruses. Findings from the Los Alamos National Laboratory indicate that it changes its genetic coding five times faster than the flu virus, which, until the appearance of HIV, was the most rapidly mutating virus known.[47] Flu vaccines must be developed or redeveloped every several years to keep abreast of viral changes (such as in the Hong Kong, the Spanish, or the swine flu). HIV may even mutate, over the decade of infection, within the infected individual, so that the same patient can harbor variant strains. Given these conditions, the production of a single, effective vaccine that will create the necessary "memory" upon which the immune system can act is improbable. A third problem stems from the fact, as noted above, that HIV is *our* virus. Few animals show any reaction at all, much less get sick, when innoculated with live virus. This means that we have no way to test (on other than human subjects) the toxicity and effectiveness of experimental vaccines. In addition, the long time period involved in HIV infection makes it difficult to collect and maintain control data such that researchers can be sure that improvements are related to use of the vaccine. Finally, certain types of vaccines, such as inactivated whole-virus vaccines, are hazardous since an imperfect manufacturing process might produce a vaccine that infects rather than confers immunity.[48] Viral-based infections have always proved difficult to counter—we have no vaccine or cure for the common cold, no universal vaccine for flu, none for any form of herpes, cytomegalovirus, Epstein-Barr, and so on through the viral pathogens that like us.[49]

REPLICATION

If cellular infection is not short-circuited, then HIV commences the intricate process of reproducing itself by using the facilities of the T4 cell. During this phase of its life cycle the virus raider is skillfully camouflaged, invisible to immune system defenders because of its integration into a human cell nucleus. However, it is vulnerable to intervention at some points, such as during the process of unloading its materials within T4 and during the process of building new boats (copies of the original) within the nucleus of the T4 cell.

The business of replicating itself is a complex enzyme-directed process that may take place long after HIV has invaded T4, or very rapidly after cellular infection. Upon entering the host cell the raiders first unload their equipment. That is, HIV destroys its own nucleus membrane and frees its genetic materials within the cell. Then the enzyme reverse transcriptase directs a restructuring of the RNA strands containing HIV's genetic information into DNA strands matching those of the human cell. These newly constituted HIV-DNA strands are then inserted into the host cell DNA, where they can be duplicated by that cell's normal division processes. In common with other members of its family, HIV cannot reproduce itself; it is at this point in its cycle that HIV's essential character as a parasite becomes clear.

The media has informed people on this aspect of HIV's life cycle more consistently than any other because, I suppose, everyone can identify with the process of reproduction and understand the significance of aborting it. AZT (3'-azido-2',3'-dideoxythymidine or Retrovir), the best known drug associated with HIV infection, is used for precisely this purpose. AZT is effective in prolonging the lives of many AIDS patients (especially if commenced early in the infection) by partially sabotaging the reproduction process. It works by fooling the enzyme (reverse transcriptase) that directs the process into incorporating a look-alike, but fake, molecular component into the viral make-up. This eventually disrupts the process and terminates replication—the molecular equivalent of throwing a monkey wrench into the works. The scientific refinement implicit in such approaches is incredible. A new drug called ddI (dideoxynosine) works to disjoint the replication process by displacing one, and only one, atom of oxygen in the chain of events necessary for replication; it is a hopeful replacement for AZT in those cases where HIV has developed an AZT tolerance or AZT is too toxic.[50] It should be noted that neither drug is cost free; both can have serious side effects in some users.[51]

RECAPITULATION

After its genetic materials are duplicated by human cell action, the materials are reorganized on RNA strands, as upon the original invading virus, and then reassembled as whole viruses in the outer portions of the host cell. If all else fails, attempts can be made to frustrate the final assembly and launch of the new viral boats (viral budding). There are several possible ways to go about this. There are at least two drugs in trial stage which, it is hoped, may confuse our raiders in the assembly and launch of their newly made boats. They are Castanospermine, which is derived from the Australian chestnut tree and Hypercin, derived from the common weed, Saint Johnswort.[52]

It is not certain, but it may be that T4 cellular death and the gradual depletion of these essential cells is partly a by-product of the assembly and launching process. While a slow production of individual HIV cells might not adversely affect the T4 cell, it does appear that an accelerated production can disrupt its membrane as newly formed HIV cells swarm out. One of the goals of therapeutic medicine is to devise means of controlling, if not stopping, the production of HIV. A slow, controlled cycle would be tantamount to a chronic but not necessarily fatal infection.

In any case, the raiders have achieved their goal, more boats and raiders. Biologically speaking, this is what both HIV and *homo sapiens* behavior are all about, the survival of the species. Properly viewed, HIV's life cycle is seen as a continuous circle of events which, after initial injection, has neither beginning nor end. We can cut into it at various points to slow the deadly wheel, but so far the only event that stops it is the host's death. Death results from one or more of the many afflictions enticed by HIV's impairment of our immune system. Acquired Immunodeficiency Syndrome is the final, the terminal human response.

PROGRESSION TO AIDS

Each of the stages in the life cycle of HIV is repeated countless times, each time doing some additional minute damage. It is common, but a bit misleading, to speak of HIV's "latency or incubation" period as though this were a period of rest or inaction.[53] What is usually being referred to is the long time lapse between infection and display of opportunistic disease symptoms. The fact is, however, that by gradually killing T4 lymphocyte cells and diminishing the effectiveness of the body's immune system, the HIV infection (that is, the aggregate action of all the viruses) does damage throughout its tenure in the human body.[54] According to a model developed at Walter Reed Hospital (Fig. 2.3) and based upon experience with military seropositives, HIV infection is seen as developing in six stages with identifiable diagnostic markers from (1) "asymptomatic seropositivity" to (6) "life-threatening opportunistic infections."[55] Initially the body's immune system does produce antibodies to the virus, but over the long run the response is inadequate. Viewing the same data in calendar stages (rather than diagnostic ones) the crossover period, during which the virus begins to gain the upper hand over the body's defense system, and symptoms begin to appear, seems to occur late in the sixth or seventh year after infection.[56] Prior to that, individuals can be quite unaware of their infection and may evidence no signs other than those that can be discerned only by lab testing (such as a gradually decreasing T4 cell count).

Another model, one that correlates the immune system's T4/CD4 cell counts with the appearance of disease symptoms, indicates that people will develop the indicator diseases necessary for an AIDS diagnosis from about the eighth year of infection. During the first six years no lasting symptoms ordinarily appear, but the cell counts drop from a healthy normal of 1000–1200 per cubic millimeter of blood to about 400. Current clinical findings indicate that this first phase, the "asymptomatic period," can be extended by low-dose AZT therapy. In the seventh year blood cell counts drop further (200–400), and some relatively mild infections, such as oral

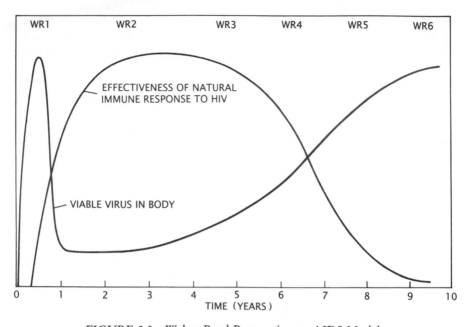

FIGURE 2.3   Walter Reed Progression-to-AIDS Model

thrush, bacterial skin infections, and shingles can appear. In the eighth year, with still lower cell counts (0–200), an HIV+ might experience serious fungal expressions (like severe athlete's foot), oral hairy leukoplakia, and tuberculosis. The ninth and subsequent years will present a variety of life-threatening infections that singly or in combination produce the final diagnosis of AIDS.[57]

In individual cases the progress from infection to a display of the AIDS symptomology is extremely variable, and little is known about why these variations exist. Age seems to be one factor. The older an individual is at the time of infection, the faster he or she progresses to AIDS.[58] Other factors that have been hypothesized as influencing the rapidity of progression are drinking, drug use, smoking, and repeated STD exposures, but there is no conclusive data on any of these usages. Personal experience is no guide in this matter. As an AIDS foundation worker I have seen glowing specimens of health, people who are careful with their diet and who exercise regularly, progress to AIDS faster than others who have clearly led a very unhealthy life. I have also seen the opposite. As in the case of cancer and other diseases, there may be genetic predispositions at work. Furthermore, the reader should keep in mind that the "average" figures used in models are just that, averages of a large number of variable, unique cases. An individual history can depart strikingly from statistical norms. For example, a counselee of mine watched his blood count drop from 900 to 526 in just two years, much faster than the average, but then the count remained at 526 for a year which, again, was not the average, expected reaction. Two other individuals enjoy reasonably good health with counts of 80 and 126 respectively, even though the standard charts and prognoses become very discouraging at these levels. As every physician with an AIDS practice can testify, the unusual is sometimes the usual in AIDS.

The average time from viral exposure to the onset of overt symptoms is seven to eight years. The median "incubation" time is thought to be from 9 to 11 years; that is, half the subjects would develop clinical AIDS in less than that time, and half in more.[59] For individuals who have a documented seven-year clinical record, approximately 36% have progressed to AIDS, another 40% have measurable deterioration in clinical markers (such as decreasing T4 cell counts), and the remainder appear asymptomatic. Assuming a normal immune system at the time of infection, the body is initially able to contain the damage of the invading virus, but over time the cumulative impact of HIV prevails. It is not known whether everyone will develop AIDS, or how long the span of progression will prove to be. But it is likely that, over a term of 15 years or so, few, if any, will escape. The final stage involves an "irreversible decline . . . marked by successive, uncontrollable opportunistic infections, progressive general deterioration and debilitation, and often deteriorating mental capacity."[60] In the final stages all that anyone can do is help the PWA die with reasonable comfort and dignity.

What is it that has developed? What is AIDS? What follows is an abbreviated statistical and clinical description. However, it needs to be said up front that no set of descriptions can convey the reality of AIDS. No one who has not heard the words, "I regret to say that your test results are positive" or who has not faced the final AIDS diagnosis, can possibly appreciate what it is like—the sinking feeling, the fear and then denial, the sense of separation from others, the final daily agony of watching your body sicken and age as though it had been suddenly switched to Fast Forward. Even those who have worked around AIDS patients cannot know. There is one book that does pierce the veil a bit—Emmanuel Dreuilhe's *Mortal Embrace: Living with AIDS*.[61] It is a brief, beautiful, and anguished work that could only have been written by someone from within the agony.

What is AIDS? First, what is it not? It is not equivalent to seropositivity, to infection with HIV. All people with AIDS will have been infected by the virus and generally test positive, but only a minority of those who test positive at any given time will have AIDS. The list of clinical ailments that are considered "indicators" of AIDS includes 20 afflictions, all of which can exist independently of AIDS, but which characteristically develop rapidly and severely in someone with an impaired immune system.[62] These afflictions are the so-called opportunistic infections, infections that take advantage of the immune system's impairment. Perhaps it would be more accurate to state that there are *groups* of opportunistic infections. For example, there are some 24 diseases associated with the central nervous system alone.

The agents of some infections are common in our environment, such as that which causes *Pneumocystis carinii* pneumonia (PCP); a majority of the readers of this book have been exposed to the fungal agent that causes it. However, the pathogen's damage potential is checked by a normal immune system.[63] On the other hand, Kaposi's sarcoma (KS) was an uncommon ailment largely confined to Mediterranean and African men prior to the HIV epidemic. Yet these two opportunistic infections are so very commonly encountered as part of the syndrome that a diagnosis is considered presumptive for AIDS. While PCP is generally not encountered outside the context of AIDS or in an otherwise immunocompromised system, KS can be. KS produces abnormal growths of blood vessels on external and internal skin membranes. It seems to be a separate epidemic disease with its own epidemiology, treatment, and impact.[64] Fortunately its incidence in the United States is declining.

Other clinical indicators for AIDS are various cytomegaloviral infections[65] such as CMV retinitis, which blinds rapidly; cryptococcal meningitis, a dangerous yeast infection; oral candidiasis (thrush), which fills the mouth and esophagus with white choking fungus; severe herpes lesions; toxoplasmosis of the brain (inflammation and irreversible brain damage), causing loss of cognitive and/or motor function; mycobacterium avium complex (MAI or MAC), which produces many symptoms including high fever, nausea, severe diarrhea, and weight loss; a mycobacterial form of tuberculosis; cryptosporidiosis (intestinal inflammation); acute renal failure;[66] and on and on and on. The full clinical list is distressingly long.

The specific opportunistic infections that afflict a given individual will vary according to a number of variables. His or her previous medical history and life style will be obvious factors. Apparently unrelated matters can affect the health of a PWA. For example, cat litter boxes and bird droppings are a fertile source of *Toxoplasma gondii*, the agent of toxoplasmosis, and therefore immunocompromised people are safer without cats and birds around. Similarly, *Mycobacteria avium* is commonly found in garden soil (no gardening), poultry, dairy products, and meats (no rare steaks). Neither of these pathogens is dangerous to anyone with a normal immune system, but both are deadly to someone with an impaired immune system. Even geographic locale can play a role. Different areas have varying concentrations of the pathogens involved. Thus in North America the fungal agent responsible for histoplasmosis is found mainly in the Mississippi Valley. Current research indicates that few of the various opportunistic infections will take firm hold until an individual's immune cell counts fall below 200.

One problem that does not appear on the list, but perhaps should, is suicide. While it is not an opportunistic infection in the ordinary sense, data nonetheless indicate an increased incidence of suicide for seropositives.[67] By the very fact of infection, the HIV+ person is set aside, isolated from others. From Biblical times into the twentieth century lepers were quarantined for, as it turned out, no good reason. Happily, we have learned, and no one in authority seriously proposes constructing HIV leprosaria. Nonetheless at the very time that a recent seroconverter most needs emotional support, he or she is least likely to get it. The fear of stigmatization is sufficient to prevent the new HIV+ person from turning to those from whom he or she would normally seek help. Frequently there is a self-quarantine process, a distancing that results from fear of public exposure and consequent loss of job, insurance, and friends. There is also the isolation that comes from the conviction that communication with "the others"—the uninfected—is futile, since no one but another HIV+ can possibly understand the shortened and difficult life ahead.[68] All this is exacerbated by a feeling of disorientation, even madness, as all the fixed points of one's life are suddenly undermined— why should one finish school, go on working, plan for the future, or continue dating a special someone? Finally, the PWA suffers a steady demoralization that results from feeling that he or she has become a pariah, a person who cannot satisfy ordinary social and sexual needs without endangering others.

Since there is at present no weapon that is lethal to the virus that is not also lethal to humans, therapy is limited to slowing its replication combined with treatment of the opportunistic infections as they appear. This secondary prophylaxis is a gradually losing game because, first, if one opportunistic infection is brought under control another can and will develop and, second, because the patient's system gradually becomes too weak to give natural support to the medical intervention. It is like trying to put out a forest fire without being able to get at the core of the blaze.

Dr. John McGowan of the AIDS program at the National Institute of Allergy and Infectious Diseases said, "We're going to have to have alphabet soup to treat this disease."[69] Workers in the field agree. There may never be a single remedy, but rather a gradually evolving potpourri of drugs, therapies, and vaccines, the exact recipe of which might vary with the patient's age, sex, general health, and display of opportunistic infections.[70] For example, it does seem that there needs to be a different "mix" for women who, for unknown reasons, develop different patterns of opportunistic infections and die faster than men.[71] The IV drug user presents his or her own set of problems. Laboratory studies indicate that HIV gets high on coke too! The virus grows three times faster in cells exposed to cocaine.[72] Similarly, pediatric cases require definition and treatment distinct from adult cases. Science is just now confronting the fact that most of the American data are derived from studies of gay men in cities like San Francisco, New York, and Chicago, while the incidence among other groups about which we know much less, such as women, is increasing rapidly.

The major weakness bedeviling the search for vaccines, more effective drugs, and better treatment protocols is the lack of knowledge about the structure and operation of HIV; with all that we have learned in such a short time, there are still glaring gaps in our understanding of how HIV works in the body, as distinct from in a test tube.[73] Basic research is fundamental to further progress. Without a thorough body of knowledge about HIV's complex relation to the human organism, science can only grope, instead of march, toward solutions.

However, even a more adequate data base does not guarantee the development of a cure in the complete, popular sense of the term. In this century it is more likely that AIDS will become a "chronic but manageable" disease, an affliction contained and managed by a much longer list of drugs than the few now approved (Table 2.2). Dr. Burton Lee, of the Sloan-Kettering Cancer Center and a member of the President's Commission on AIDS, put the matter this way: "There's no pie in the sky with AIDS. The sad fact is that medicine has never cured a viral disease, and AIDS is caused by an exceptionally complicated retrovirus." No one should expect a quick fix.

Notes

1. Apart from molecular-biological variations, there seem to be two principal differences between HIV I and HIV II. First, HIV II is much less widespread. While some infections have been isolated in the United States, it is found mainly in western Africa. Second, it progresses to AIDS even more slowly than HIV I. Both are deadly.
2. Paul Cotton, "HIV Genes Overlap with Ours," *Medical World News*, March 14, 1988, p. 38. Emmanuel Dreuilhe, *Mortal Embrace: Living with AIDS* (New York: Hill and Wang, 1988).
3. See the review of theories in Jad Adams, *AIDS: the HIV Myth* (New York: St. Martin's Press, 1989), Chap. 7.
4. On the biologic origin of HIV, see: Robert C. Gallo, "The AIDS Virus, Part II," *Scientific American*, January 1987, p. 56; Max Essex and Phyllis J. Kanki, "The Origins of the AIDS Virus," *Scientific American*, October 1988, pp. 64–71; Max Essex, "Origins of AIDS," in Vincent T. DeVita *et al.* (eds.), *AIDS, Etiology,*

TABLE 2.2   Approved Medicines

Drug Name	Utilization	Company
Bactrin (Trimethoprim & sulfamethoazole	*Pneumocystis carinii* pneumonia treatment	Hoffman-LaRoche, NJ
Cytovene (Ganciclovir IV)	Cytomegalovirus retinitis treatment	Syntex, Palo Alto, CA
Daraprim (Pyrimenthamine)	Toxoplasmosis treatment	Burroughs Wellcome, NC
Diflucan (Fluconazole)	Cryptococcal meningitis & candidiasis treatment	Pfizer, NY
Intron A (Interferon-alpha 2b)	Kaposi's sarcoma treatment	Schering-Plough, NJ
Nebupent (Aerosol pentamidine isethionate)	PCP prophylaxis	LyphoMed, IL
Pentam 300	PCP treatment	LyphoMed
Retrovir (Zidovudine, AZT)	AIDS treatment	Burroughs Wellcome
Roferon A	Kaposi's sarcoma	Hoffman-LaRoche
Septra Trimethroprim & suphpamethazole)	PCP treatment	Burroughs Wellcome

Source: From information presented by the Pharmaceutical Manufacturers Association in cooperation with the American Foundation for AIDS Research and the Food and Drug Administration. FDA approved drugs through February 10, 1990.

Diagnosis, Treatment, and Prevention (New York: J. B. Lippincott Co., 1988). See also the good summary in Professor A. Karpas' letter to *Nature*, December 13, 1990, p. 578.

5. Eve K. Nichols, *Mobilizing against AIDS*, rev. ed. (Washington, DC: Institute of Medicine, National Academy of Sciences, 1989), p. 109.

6. See the chilling demographic projections of R. M. Anderson and the Parasite Epidemiology Research Group, Department of Pure and Applied Biology, Imperial College, London University. R. M. Anderson *et al.*, "The Impact of the Spread of HIV on Population Growth and Age Structure in Developing Countries," in Alan F. Fleming *et al.* (eds.), *The Global Impact of AIDS: Proceedings of the First International Conference on the Global Impact of AIDS.* Cospon-

sored by the World Health Organization and the London School of Hygiene and Tropical Medicine, London, March 8–10, 1988 (New York: Alan R. Liss, 1988), Chapter 12.

7. It should be noted that while the majority of the scientific establishment seems to support the position that HIV is the causative agent in AIDS, there is a minority position. Dr. Peter H. Duesberg, Professor of Molecular Biology, University of California at Berkeley, is a major protagonist of another view which denies that HIV is that agent. Dr. Duesberg published his challenge to conventional HIV theory in the February 1989 issue of the *Proceedings of the National Academy of Sciences* ("Human Immunodeficiency Virus and Acquired Immunodeficiency Syndrome: Correlation but not Causation"). Dr. Duesberg contends that AIDS is caused by a combination of (1) "chronic promiscuous male homosexual activity," (2) "parasitic infection," (3) malnutrition, and (4) narcotic toxins. See the interesting comment in *Science* (February 10, 1989, p. 733) on the fight between Duesberg and the National Academy. The minority position is reviewed in Adams, *AIDS: The HIV Myth*. Another major research scientist whose work raises questions about the role of HIV is Dr. Shyh-Ching Lo, who is the head of the AIDS pathology division of the Armed Forces Institute of Pathology's Molecular Pathobiology Laboratory. See his study in the *American Journal of Tropical Medicine Hygiene* 40 (1989): 213–226, 399–409. There is also the possibility that a mycoplasma organism is involved in the development of the syndrome. Mycoplasmas are the smallest known organisms which, unlike viruses, have the ability to reproduce themselves. They occupy a biological niche someplace between bacteria and viruses. A group of scientists met in San Antonio in December 1989 to explore this possibility. *San Antonio Express-News*, December 9, 1989, p. 14a. Brant Mittler, "Behold, AIDS Research Behind Closed Doors," *Medical Tribune*, February 8, 1990. Dr. Luc Montagnier of France, whose team discovered HIV, gave some support to the view that mycoplasmas may be co-factors in statements at the Sixth International Conference on AIDS, San Francisco, July 1990. "AIDS Drugs—Coming, but Not Here," *Science*, April 21, 1990, p. 287.

8. An international controversy, ultimately involving the presidents of France and the United States, developed over who discovered what and when. National and professional pride, as well as valuable patent rights, were involved in this rather degrading conclusion to a notable scientific achievement. Good summaries can be read in: *Journal of the American Medical Association (JAMA)*, December 25, 1987, pp. 3482–87; and *Chicago Tribune*, November 19, 1989. The *Tribune* ran an extraordinary pair of articles by investigative reporter John Crewdson on this controversy. See also: "The French Connection, II: An International AIDS Dispute Is Reborn," *Newsweek*, April 2, 1990, p. 65. In October 1990 the National Institutes of Health announced that they were undertaking a full-scale investigation of "possible misconduct" (that is, copying the French discoveries rather than independently developing them) in Dr. Gallo's laboratory at the National Cancer Institute.

9. The American figure is very "soft" and very debatable. It was derived, at the 1986 Coolfont Planning Conference, by extrapolating from the assumed number of homosexuals in the United States (as projected from the Kinsey research of the 1940s). At that time there were about 30,000 cases reported. It did not take into consideration other transmission modes like IV drug use. In 1989 California epidemiologists were stating that there might be over 2 million infected in that

state alone. It is more than possible that an accurate national survey would more than triple the old 1.5 million guesstimate. The "official" estimate stated by the Federal Centers for Disease Control in 1990 is 1 million.

10. T4 and CD4 are different names for the same molecular receptor. HIV is capable of attaching to and infecting monocytes/macrophages, using them for transportation throughout the body, including the brain and central nervous system. HIV has also been isolated in the Langerhans cells of the skin.

11. P. C. Fox, *et al.*, "Saliva Inhibits HIV-1 Infectivity," *Journal of the American Dental Association*, 116, no. 6 (1988): 635–37. A. C. Varrusio, *et al.*, "Risk of Transmission of the Human Immunodeficiency Virus to Health Care Workers Exposed to HIV-Infected Patients: A Review," *Journal of the American Dental Association*, 118, no. 3 (1989): 229–342.

12. Mangalasseril & Markham, "Role of Human T Lymphotropic Retrovirus in Leukemia and AIDS," in Gary P. Wormser *et al.* (eds.), *AIDS: Acquired Immune Deficiency Syndrome* (Park Ridge, NJ: Noyes 1987), p. 219.

13. HIV 2 is the most commonly known. The first reported infection by this agent in the United States was in 1987. Since then 16 additional cases have been found. "AIDS Update of Experimental Therapies," *Health Info-Com Network Newsletter*, May 16, 1990. James Brooke, "Virus Discoveries," *New York Times*, February 28, 1988, p. 12.

14. For a much more extensive description of the immune system and the molecular biology of the virus, but one that is still geared to the nonbiologist, see Mary Catherine Bateson and Richard Goldsby, *Thinking AIDS* (Addison-Wesley, 1988), Chaps. 3–6; or William B. Johnson and Kevin R. Hopkins, *The Catastrophe Ahead, AIDS and the Case for a New Public Policy* (New York: Praeger, 1990), Chap. 6. A more technical and extended description, but still accessible to the nonbiologist, can be read in Nichols, *Mobilizing against AIDS* Chap. 5. For those interested in professional descriptions of HIV's life cycle, I suggest William A. Haseltine and Flossie Wong-Staal, "The Molecular Biology of the AIDS Virus," and Robert Yarchoan, Hiroaki Mitsuya, and Samuel Broder, "AIDS Therapies," *Scientific American*, October 1988; Vincent T. DeVita *et al.*, *AIDS, Etiology, Diagnosis, Treatment, and Prevention*, 2nd ed. (New York: J. B. Lippincott, 1988), Chaps. 2 and 5.

15. It is likely that virus-infected cells, rather than free virus, are the principal transmitting mechanism. Jay Levy, *JAMA*, May 27, 1988, p. 3037.

16. For technical descriptions see: Wormser, *AIDS*, Chaps. 9, 11; Institute of Medicine, National Academy of Sciences, *Confronting AIDS: Directions for Public Health Care and Research* (National Academy Press, 1986), Chap. 6; Anthony Fauci, "The Human Immunodeficiency Virus: Infectivity and Mechanisms of Pathogenesis," *Science* 239: 617–621. For popularized technical versions see: William A. Haseltine and Flossie Wong-Staal, "Molecular Biology of the AIDS Virus"; Jonathan Weber and Robin A. Weiss, "HIV Infection: The Cellular Picture," *Scientific American*, October 1988.

17. See Alan R. Lifson, "Do Alternate Modes of Transmission of HIV Exist?" *JAMA*, March 4, 1988, p. 1353.

18. U.S. Department of Public Health and Human Services, Public Health Service, Centers for Disease Control, *Morbidity and Mortality Weekly Report. Supplement: Recommendations for Prevention of HIV Transmission in Health-Care Settings* (Washington, D.C., 1987). On the development of new types of surgical gloving, see *Medical Tribune*, March 8, 1990, p. 7.

19. Many more have been exposed. Hard, reliable data are difficult to come by in this area because the virus may not evidence itself in tests until long after the presumed needle-stick incident. It is difficult to establish clear cause and effect. "Why Fear Persists: Health Care Professionals and AIDS," *JAMA*, December 16, 1988, p. 3481. Ruthanne Marcus, "Surveillance of Health Care Workers Exposed to Blood from Patients Infected with the Human Immunodeficiency Virus," *N. Engl. J. Med.*, October 27, 1988, pp. 1118–19.

20. *JAMA*, November 7, 1990. See the excellent special report by Elisabeth Rosenthal, "Practice of Medicine Is Changing under Specter of the AIDS Virus," *New York Times*, November 11, 1990, p. A1.

21. The data supporting this recommendation are inconclusive, but no real test of it is possible since it would entail the death of the physician. Dr. Marcus A. Conant made the recommendation at the annual meeting of the American Academy of Dermatology. See "HIV, Hepatitis Continue to Pose Major Risks for Health Workers," *Internal Medicine News*, January 15–31, 1990, p. 1.

22. Sar Staver, "One in 250 HIV-Infected Sticks Transmits the Virus—Studies," *American Medical News*, January 13, 1989, pp. 19–20. And see interview with Dr. Lorraine Day, who resigned as Chief of Orthopedic Surgery at San Francisco General Hospital to protest inadequate medical and hospital administrative response to the hazards of the operating room. *New Dimensions*, March 1990, pp. 36–40.

23. The *New York Times* cites the Soviet magazine *Ogonyok*, which stated that in 1988 the Soviet Union produced only 7 million disposable syringes a year against an estimated need of 6 billion, and 200 million condoms against a need of 1 billion. John F. Burns, "Outbreak of AIDS Triples: Testing in a Soviet City," *New York Times*, National Section, February 5, 1989.

24. This tragic story was told by Dr. Vladimir Pokrovsky, the representative of the Soviet Union at the Fifth International Conference on AIDS, which met in Montreal in June 1989. See *New York Times*, June 3, 1989. The Soviet Union has enacted new legislation making multiple uses of syringes and other dangerous practices subject to criminal prosecution. However, the nation is still far from producing adequate supplies of antiseptic and disposable equipment.

25. *Ogonyok*, cited in *Health InfoCom Newsletter*, April 20–22, 1990. And see also *Nature*, June 14, 1990, which contains a commentary on some official Soviet reports of the possibility of great increases in the incidence of AIDS.

26. Summary in "Transfusion-Transmitted AIDS Reassessed," (editorial), *JAMA*, 318, no. 8: 511.

27. Randy Shilts, *And the Band Played On* (New York: St. Martin's Press, 1987), relates this story in detail. Also see John W. Ward, "Tranfusion of HIV by Blood Transfusions Screened as Negative for the HIV Antibody," and Thomas F. Zuck, "Transfusion-Transmitted AIDS Reassessed," *N. Engl. J. Med.*, February 25, 1988, pp. 473, 511.

28. *Congressional Quarterly*, August 18, 1990, p. 2685.

29. See the summary article, Sandra Blakeslee, "Blood Banks Facing Hundreds of AIDS Suits," *New York Times*, Health Section, April 27, 1989, p. 24. Janice Somerville, "AIDS Related Suits," *American Medical News*, February 17, 1989. The problem is not confined to the United States. *The Melbourne Star Observer*, September 8, 1989, reported that hundreds of Australian hemophiliacs may sue the Red Cross blood bank for receiving contaminated blood-clotting agents between 1983 and 1985. The estimates are that one-fourth of Australia's hemophiliacs are infected.

30. See John W. Ward *et al.*, "Transmission of Human Immunodeficiency Virus by Blood Transfusions Screened as Negative for HIV Antibody," *N. Engl. J. Med.*, February 25, 1988, pp. 473–77. The risk of transmitting HIV through transfusion of screened blood is calculated as 1:153,000 to 1:200,000. See *N. Engl. J. Med.*, March 22, 1990, p. 850. There is considerable argument in the professional literature about the possibility of testing negative on the ELISA or Western blot while being infected with the virus. There is also controversy about how long a person can be infected without testing positive in the standard tests. Very sophisticated, expensive, and time-consuming tests approach 100% accuracy, but are too elaborate to be used in mass operations like blood plasma collection. The Ryan White Comprehensive AIDS Act of 1990 authorized a special study running from 1991 through 1995 as well as Federal services to help protect the blood supply.

31. "Special Report: How Safe Is Our Blood Supply?" *Reader's Digest*, July 1988, pp. 37–44. This report points out that there have been 13 cases of transfusion AIDS since 1985, when screening was finally implemented.

32. "New York Won't Tell Doctors with AIDS to Inform Patients," *New York Times*, January 19, 1990, p. A1. See also "AIDS and the Privacy of Doctors: A Touchy Issue at Bellevue," *New York Times*, January 28, 1991, p. A15; Sari Staver, "Government Guidelines Coming Soon on Managing HIV-Infected Health Care Workers," *American Medical News*, December 28, 1990, p. 3, and "HIV Infected Doctors Should Tell Patients, Stop Surgery—AMA," *American Medical News*, February 4, 1991, p. 1.

33. David Hill, "HIV Infection Following Motor Vehicle Trauma in Central Africa," *JAMA*, June 9, 1989, p. 3282.

34. *Washington HIV News* 1, no. 4 (January 1990).

35. For a review of the situation see Kristin White, "Treating Pediatric AIDS," *AIDS Patient Care* 1, no. 1, (September 1987): 5–13. Gwendolyn Scott *et al.*, "Survival of Children with Perinatally Acquired Human Immunodeficiency Virus Type 1 Infection," *N. Engl. J. Med.*, January 1990, pp. 1791–96.

36. "Aids Boarder Babies Pose Financial and Logistical Problems," *AIDS ALERT* 3, no. 6 (June 1988): 97–102.

37. See "Researchers Gain in Mapping How AIDS Virus Enters Cells," *New York Times*, December 29, 1990, p. A1.

38. For a review see Fred T. Valentine, "Pathogenesis of the Immunological Deficiencies Caused by Infection with the Human Immunodeficiency Virus," *Seminars in Oncology* 17, no. 3 (June 1990): 321–334.

39. Trials are under way on a number of drugs trying this approach. AL-721, a promising toxin, is under development now. It is a poisonous product of the *Pseudomonas* bacteria that can attach and destroy cells infected with HIV. It is hoped that it can be used to control the spread of the virus, although it is not a cure. See Gina Kolata, "Scientists Modify Powerful Toxic to Combat Spread of AIDS Virus," *New York Times*, October 14, 1988.

40. Robert W. Finbert *et al.*, "Prevention of HIV-1 Infection and Preservation of CD4 function by the binding of CPFs to gp120," *Science*, July 20, 1990, p. 287.

41. For an excellent summary of the prospects and problems see "Vaccine Development," in *AIDS Summary: In-Depth Review & Update* (Philadelphia, PA: Philadelphia Sciences Group Publications, March 1989).

42. "Test of a Vaccine on Monkeys Offers New Hope in AIDS Fight," *New York Times*, December 8, 1989, p. 1.

43. Dr. Ronald Derosiers of the New England Regional Primate Center, quoted in

John Capri, "The AIDS Vaccine Front Is Expanding," *Medical Tribune*, March 8, 1990, p. 7.

44. Maurice R. Hilleman, "Conclusions: In Pursuit of an AIDS Virus Vaccine," in Jay A. Levy (ed.), *AIDS, Pathogenesis and Treatment* (New York: Marcel Dekker, 1989), p. 609.

45. *CDC AIDS Weekly*, (Atlanta, GA: Charles Henderson, publ.), November 7, 1988, p. 3.

46. The term "vaccine development," in the singular, is somewhat misleading. Actually, research is under way on many different types of vaccines, each with its own set of problems and potentials. There are inactivated, attenuated live, recombinant DNA, hybrid virus, synthesized polypeptide, and anti-idiotype vaccines.

47. See Bradley D. Preston *et al.*, "Fidelity of HIV-1 Reverse Transcriptase," *Science*, November 25, 1988, p. 1168. The findings are that HIV's extensive genetic variation and rapid evolution are due to the high "error" rate of reverse transcriptase, the enzyme that directs part of the replication process. The authors use the term "hypermutability."

48. See the report on the Third Annual International Conference on Advances in AIDS Vaccine Development (sponsored by NIAID), in *Science*, October 12, 1990.

49. Effective antiviral vaccines have been developed against vaccinia, poliovirus, measles, mumps, rubella, yellow fever, influenza, rabies, and hepatitis B.

50. See Nichols, *Mobilizing against AIDS*, Chap. 7, for a brief coverage of the various agents now in testing and trial stages.

51. For the first long-term studies on ddI see R. Yarchoan *et al.*, "Long-Term Toxicity/Activity Profile of 2,3′-Dideoxyinosine in AIDS or AIDS-Related Complex," *The Lancet*, September 1, 1990.

52. "AIDS Drugs—Coming, but Not Here," *Science*, April 21, 1990, p. 287.

53. It is not known why the period of so-called latency is as long as it is. The authors of an interesting attempt to model viral development or evolution after infection hypothesize that "the most important single factor leading to breakdown of immune control of HIV is the increase in the diversity of the virus." Charles R. M. Bangham and Andrew J. McMichael, "Why the Long Latent Period," *Nature*, November 29, 1990.

54. David Ho *et al.*, "Quantitation of Human Immunodeficiency Virus, Type 1 in Blood of Infected Person," *N. Engl. J. Med.*, December 14, 1989, p. 1621.

55. For a description of the Walter Reed system see Appendix C in *Report of the Presidential Commission on the Human Immunodeficiency Virus*, June 24, 1988.

56. Robert Redfield and Donald Burke, "HIV Infection: The Clinical Picture," *Scientific American*, October 1988, pp. 93–98. This article explains the classification system developed by the authors. Their system delineates "stages" in the progression to AIDS. They are both scientists at Walter Reed Army Institute of Research, Washington, DC. Redfield is chief of the retrovirology section, Burke is chief of the Department of Virus Diseases at the Institute of Research. Another, perhaps more accurate, method of tracking the progression is through CD4 cell counts. See K. B. MacDonnell *et al.*, "Prognostic Usefulness of the Walter Reed Staging Classification for HIV Infection," *Journal of Acquired Immune Deficiency Syndromes* (1988): 367–374.

57. See the excellent review article by John Mills and Henry Masur, "AIDS-Related Infections," *Scientific American*, August 1990, p. 50.

58. Gina Kolata, "Researchers Link Speed of AIDS Development to Age," *New York Times*, National, May 21, 1989.
59. The 11-year estimate is documented by George F. Lemp, *et al.*, "Projections of AIDS Morbidity and Mortality in San Francisco," *JAMA*, March 16, 1990. The 10-year figure is the result of the San Francisco Department of Health study. Peter Bacchetti and Andrew Moss, "AIDS Incubation Time," *Nature*, March 16, 1988, pp. 251–53. Gina Kolata, "AIDS Incubation Time Often Exceeds 9 Years," *New York Times*, Health, March 16, 1989, p. 19.
60. Donald I. Abrams, Jeanee Parker-Martin, and Kenneth Unger, "AIDS: Caring for the Dying Patient," *Patient Care*, November 30, 1989, p. 22 *et seq.*
61. Emmanuel Dreuilhe, *Mortal Embrace, Living with AIDS* (New York: Hill and Wang, 1988).
62. For a technical but still accessible description of the entire range of infections see Gifford Leoung and John Mills (eds.), *Opportunistic Infections in Patients with the Acquired Immunodeficiency Syndrome* (New York: Marcel Dekker, 1989).
63. For the full range of pulmonary complications see John F. Murray and John Mills, "Pulmonary Infectious Complications of Human Immunodeficiency Virus Infection" (in 2 parts), *American Review of Respiratory Diseases*, 141 (1990).
64. "KS Is Not Cancer; Is It Also Not AIDS?" *AIDS Treatment News*, March 16, 1990, and the references cited there. Recent research indicates that certain of the HIV cell proteins have the effect of greatly stimulating KS cells into an aggressive growth. But KS and HIV infection can exist independently of one another.
65. Matthew Stenger (ed.), *The Management of HIV-Related Cytomegalovirus Infections.* Highlights of a symposium on current therapies and future strategies in the management of CMV infections held prior to the Sixth International Conference on AIDS, San Francisco, June 1990. Newsletter published by Professional Healthcare Communications (ProHealth), One Lombard St., San Francisco, CA 94111. Also distributed as *AIDS Clinical Update*, October 1, 1990, by New York's Gay Men's Health Crisis.
66. Jacques J. Bourgoignie, "Renal Complications of Human Immunodeficiency Virus Type 1," *Kidney International (Nephrology Forum)* 37 (1990): 1571–84.
67. Peter M. Marzuk *et al.*, "Increased Risk of Suicide in Persons with AIDS," *JAMA*, March 4, 1988, pp. 1333–42. See also the Associated Press feature article that appeared in the first week of July 1990 in which the director of an AIDS support group in Vancouver admitted that he had helped patients take their lives by leaving fatal overdoses within reach. *San Antonio Express-News*, July 5, 1990, p. 8e. How much assisted and unassisted suicide goes on is probably impossible to estimate with any degree of accuracy. But that it does occur is unquestionable.
68. See on this aspect Dreuilhe, *Mortal Embrace*.
69. *Science*, April 21, 1990, p. 287.
70. See "New Eclecticism Approach to AIDS," *American Medical News*, September 23/30, 1988.
71. "Women with AIDS Seen Dying Faster," *New York Times*, October 19, 1987, reporting the research of Dr. Margaret Fischl of the University of Miami. There are some clues indicating that this effect is due to the differences in male-female hormonal components, see John S. James, "DHEA, Mystery AIDS Treatment," *AIDS Treatment News*, January 15, 1988. The substance involved in this new experimental treatment is dehydroepiandrosterone, which is a steroid secreted by the adrenal gland and is closely related to the male hormone, testosterone.

72. *Health InfoCom Medical News*, October 22–24, 1990.
73. "Molecule X: The Other Key to HIV?" *New Scientist*, July 7, 1990, p. 26. The phrase "glaring gaps" is a quote from Dr. Anthony Fauci, head of National Institute of Allergy and Infectious Diseases, National Institutes of Health.

3

===

Then and Now: The Bubonic Plague and AIDS

LAUNCHING AN EPIDEMIC

Every living thing has a territory in which it evolved and from which it emerged to face the world, a home base on this planet. There are Bengal tigers, American bison, and unending hosts of butterflies, salmon, birds, whales and caribou that annually migrate back to their point of origin. We humans, who now cover the Earth, apparently are descendants of ancient hominids who evolved in places like the Olduvai Basin of central Africa's Great Rift Valley millions of years ago. Evidence of our dispersal is buried in the dirt of archaeological sites; painted on cave walls; incised on clay tablets; written on papyri, manuscripts, books, and now the electronic impulses of the computer. We call it the spread of human culture and civilization.

It is the same for the invisible empire of microbes that prey upon us. Some home-base areas, like India's Ganges River Valley, China's Yellow River Valley, and equatorial Africa and America, seem to have been designed as natural kitchens serving endless varieties of bacteria, plasmodia, viruses, protozoa, and fungi. These are areas where disease pathogens develop and are endemic. They serve as the initial staging areas for epidemics. To borrow an elegant phrase from epidemiology, they are the original geographic foci of endemicity. Sailors in the nineteenth century British navy had a more pointed expression: they referred to a tour of duty off the coast of equatorial Africa as the "coffin cruise." Having no independent means of locomotion, microbes generally stay home—unless, of course, they encounter people. Then, if conditions are right, rapid dispersal is possible. We call this unwanted event an epidemic.

Like human cultures, epidemics also leave their record, in burial grounds across the world. Records state that 20,000 per day perished in the Great

43

Plague of which Bishop Cyprian wrote in the third century. The bubonic plague of 1347–1350 killed from 17 million to 28 million, and in the 400 years of revisitations (1340–1740s), perhaps a total of 50 million. Ninety million Central and South American Indians died from waves of smallpox, measles, typhus, and flu introduced by the Spanish after 1520.[1] Seven million succumbed to cholera in 1910–1920, and another 10 million to 20 million died in the 1917 flu epidemic. Today we have perhaps 10,000,000 individuals infected with HIV. The World Health Organization predicts that this will increase to between 50 million and 100 million by 1995. For some microbes, but by no means all, and certainly not HIV, we have established a degree of effective medical treatment, control, and containment. We have eliminated only smallpox.

Seen as events of possibly global extent, epidemics or pandemics are the product of many interacting variables. Like earthquakes, volcanic eruptions, and great storms, their complexity is mind-boggling.[2] There are three major groups of variables: (1) the characteristics of the specific microbe, (2) the characteristics of potential hosts and (3) environmental conditions.

THE ETIOLOGIC AGENT

In the beginning there must be a bug. What are its characteristics, its operating parameters? Is it endemic to some remote area, like the deadly Ebola fever, or happily residing in a major population center, like cholera or dysentery in Calcutta? Does it pass part of its life cycle in the essential water supply like schistosomiasis? Is it a relatively rare fungus, or a common microorganism that surrounds us—like that which produces *Pneumocystis carinii* pneumonia in PWAs? Does it have a symbiotic, nondestructive relationship to its carrier like that of the malaria plasmodia to their carrier mosquitoes, or might it kill its host as does the smallpox virus? What is its virulence? Does it sicken (like food poisoning from the salmonella virus lurking everywhere), produce long-term debilitation (like malaria), or kill? And if it kills, what is the (natural or untreated) mortality rate—45% as in the bubonic plague or 100% as is so far the case with AIDS?

THE HOST

Next, there must be a host—or, more accurately, hosts, for one infection does not an epidemic make! HIV has been in the United States at least since the early 1960s, but we date the epidemic from 1981. In St. Louis, Missouri, in 1969, a young man named Robert died of what now appears to have been AIDS. He had never been out of the country, and was probably infected with HIV in the early to mid-1960s. But at the time his case was an isolated, unexplained infection, and, if it was passed on, the numbers were so small as to escape notice.[3] Not only must there be many potential hosts, but they should be living in close proximity. Epidemics thrive only if there is sufficient density of population for the contagion to be passed on. At minimum, the time/space factors must be within the parameters established by the natural infectivity of the bug. To put it another way, in order to keep an infection going, the number of newly infected people added to the existing reservoir of infected people must balance or exceed the number dropping out through recovery or death. Otherwise the epidemic sputters out like a fire that has finally consumed all its fuel. During the Middle Ages entire religious houses were destroyed simply because the men and women, living in closed and close communities, presented ideal transmission conditions for the plague bacillus. Today we have various urban subenvironments that are conducive to the spread of many transmissible pathogens, including HIV. Heterosexual and homosexual sex emporia, drug "shooting galleries," penitentiaries, and college dormitories all present better-than-average transmission environments. Dispersed agricultural populations are not generally subject to epidemics, although individual infections can and do occur.[4] Epidemics, at least epidemics before AIDS, have been urban, metropolitan events.[5]

There are other relevant host characteristics. The impact of an epidemic will vary with the demographic structure of the host population; adult/child, age group, gender group, and other kinds of ratios are very important. Other significant factors are the overall nutrition and health of the population, the prevalence of other debilitating afflictions, and whether or not the target population has, through previous visitations, built up some natural immunity.

THE SETTING

There are many environmental factors that affect the initiation, duration, and severity of an epidemic. For example, the flea that carries bubonic plague prefers ground-nesting rodents; the rodents (like the California ground squirrel), in turn, prefer semi-arid grasslands, which provide nesting sites and grain foods. Consequently, in ordinary circumstances the spread of the microbe will be limited by the availability of rodents which, in turn, is limited by the availability of territory and food. It is estimated that the plague bacillus could not travel more than ten miles per year and would eventually be stopped as its carrier rat encountered barriers specific to it, such as the end of the grasslands. Climate, weather, and season are other factors of significance. It can get too cold for the malarial mosquito to function, or it can be the wrong season for a virus. When I was a young man, back in the 1940s, all parents dreaded the onset of the spring and summer polio season but were unconcerned the rest of the year.

The above is just minimally suggestive of the variables involved in determining whether or not epidemic possibilities exist. The actual matrix would differ with each microbe in its cultural and environmental context. It can be likened, I think, to the definition of critical mass in assessing the possibilities of nuclear meltdown/explosion, although judging whether or not all relevant factors are in proper relation to trigger an epidemic is infinitely more complex and problematic. Still, when that point is reached disaster strikes.

Before the age of AIDS the word "epidemic" for most people evoked images of either Biblical events or the bubonic plague of the fourteenth century. But it is really the latter, the Black Death, that is our archetype epidemic; it has been *THE EPIDEMIC* of Western cultural memory. It is enshrined in our literature, from Boccaccio's *Decameron* (1350) to Camus' *The Plague* (1947), and its devastation helped bring about sea changes in the culture to which we all are heir. Notwithstanding the bubonic plague's significance, AIDS may well become the archetype epidemic for future generations. A comparison is in order.

The Global Spread of Bubonic Plague

The microbe that causes the bubonic plague is called *Yersinia pestis*. It is a microscopic, round-headed bacillus that infests the nests of ground-burrowing rodents such as the wild gerbil, the Asian marmot, and the California ground squirrel. The microbe's ancient and original home bases seem to have been central Asia and southern Africa, but today it is found in all semi-arid grassland areas that are the natural habitat of the host rodent population. For example, today California, New Mexico, and west Texas (which had a 1987–1988 episode) are major centers of endemicity.[6] As mentioned before, young rodents leaving the nest can carry the bacillus limited distances and thereby over many, many generations are able to gradually spread the infection throughout their habitat. The agent by which the bacillus is transferred from rodent to rodent is the rat flea, which gets a stomach full of the bacillus when drawing blood. The bacilli then multiply in the flea's digestive tract until they are disgorged into the bloodstream of a new rodent-host. There are over 2000 varieties of fleas, of which about 120 can transmit the deadly microbe. The rodent host dies from the infection and the flea is forced to find a new host; it much prefers a rat, but there are a few that, in a pinch, will transfer to a passing human.

A human can be afflicted with one of three varieties: (1) the standard form, which produces the classic symptoms of discolored swellings, especially in the armpit and groin areas, a putrid body smell, a spastic jerkiness of action, and a 45% chance of death within three days; (2) the rarer septicemic form, which results from an extra-large disgorging of bacilli by the flea. Death follows within a few hours of infection, so rapidly that no symptoms have time to develop; and finally (3) the pneumonic form, in which the bacillus is transferred from human to human through sneezes and coughs. Like the septicemic form, this is also rapidly fatal. One of the classic forewarnings of bubonic plague was and is a visible abundance of dead rodents and, less visibly, their deadly orphaned fleas.[7] But how did the microbe move out from its home base ultimately to infect Europe, Asia, and the Americas in wave after wave of disastrous epidemics from before the time of Christ into the twentieth century?[8]

The flea hitchhiked from its original home in central Asia on the great trade routes of the ancient world. China and the Mediterranean world were linked by caravan routes that ran between the eastern Mediterranean trading centers of Istanbul, Tyre, Antioch, Damascus, Baghdad, and Niniveh in the west to Lanzhou and Zian of China in the east. From 500 B.C. the network of caravan routes gradually became more established, safer, and more heavily used. The last links of what became known as the Silk Roads were forged by the Han Emperor Wu, who in the second century B.C. sought to extend China's influence to the West by regularizing trade with the Middle East. Two of these ancient commercial highways are of special interest. One commenced at Tyre, Antioch, and Damascus and proceeded via Hamadan and Tehran to Samarkand and Tashkent in what is now the Soviet Union. There it linked with another, the Steppe Route, which started at Istanbul, went to Tbilisi (now in Soviet Georgia), looped over the northern shores of the Caspian Sea, and then proceeded through the steppes of central Asia to Tashkent. The joined routes then skirted the northern foothills of the Himalayas, crossed over mountain passes and dropped into Xinjiang, the northwestern-most province of China. These routes of the ancient world allowed East and West to exchange ideas and goods, but they also exposed both the Oriental and Occidental populations to recurring epidemics because they crossed through the central Asian home bases of *Y. pestis*. When caravans dumped their bales of Chinese silk for the clothing of the Mediterranean upper classes they also deposited rats and fleas. The bacillus was then spread, hopscotch-like, by trading vessels sailing from seaport to seaport around the periphery of the Mediterranean. The epidemics that ensued were the unintended by-product of commercial intercourse.

Ironically, one of the most characteristic of human activities—and the one we all depend upon to enrich our material lives—was and is the single most important method of spreading deadly microbes. The irony is compounded by the fact that war, another of our major activities, is second only to commerce as an engine spreading pestilence throughout the world. The infamous Black Death, the plague of the 1340s that prostrated Europe, may have commenced with the siege of the Black Sea port of Kaffa in December 1346 by horse-mounted Tartar troops. The chroniclers of the siege of Kaffa relate that the Tartar chieftain catapulted plague-ridden bodies from his troops over the walls of Kaffa to spread disease and force the city to capitulate. This may be the first recorded instance of germ warfare.[9] In any case, within two years the plague had spread from its point of origin to England and all Europe. Transport was provided by coastal vessels carrying goods from one port city to another and, of course, from there to inland centers like Paris, where so many people died that wolves moved into the city.

The plague's spread was temporarily halted in England, Europe, and Asia. From the fourteenth through the seventeenth centuries it visited and revisited England, the Continent, and the Mediterranean, but did not move to other continents. European folklore linked rats, death and evil, a still riveting combination in our cultural and literary imagination; think of the vampire Nosferatu, nightmare of God, stalking the land accompanied by his retinue of plague-bearing rats. And everyone knows the tale of the Pied Piper. The town elders of Hamelin hired him to protect the town and its children from rats. He did so. When they reneged the Piper took all the children as payment. The plague would have taken only half. Perhaps there is a lesson for today's leaders in this tale of political dishonor.

The behavioral engines of its spread through the seventeenth century had been commerce and war, and the technology that made it possible were the caravan and the short-hop coastal sailing vessel. It requires some stretch of the space-travelling twentieth-century imagination to recapture the technological innovations the transcontinental caravan and the coastal sailing vessel represented in their time. The caravan was a marvel of logistic organization, long-range planning, and land navigation through uncharted wilderness. It required great sums of risk capital, the cooperation and support of all political systems along the route, and no small amount of good luck. Similarly, the coastal trading vessel made feasible the movement of bulky commodities that would have defied economic land transport, particularly along the complex indented northern coast of the Mediterranean from Turkey to Spain. Both of these modes operated within time frames that met the biologic requirements of transmitting the plague. A coastal vessel could load goods with its accompanying rats/fleas and discharge them elsewhere before everyone on board became infected and died. A voyage of too long duration simply meant that an epidemic contained on board would sputter out before reaching port; there were many instances of ships drifting ashore with all rats and all hands dead. Only the fleas would be left on the "ghost ships" of lore.

Before *Y. Pestis* could spread to the New World, a major step in transport technology had to be made, one that would shorten the passage time. This came in the late nineteenth century with the development of the transoceanic steamship. Along with the railroad, it ushered in the age of mass movement of people and goods and the rapid dispersal of epidemic agents. It made possible the spread of the bubonic plague to every spot on the globe which had been, up to that time, blessedly free of it. The steamship arrival of the bubonic plague in California, probably from Asian ports, is generally dated around the turn of the twentieth century. In March 1900 San Francisco had its first panicky brush with the Black Death after the body of a Chinese man, dead from plague, was found in the basement of a Chinatown hotel. The board of health, backed by the mayor, cordoned and quarantined twelve square blocks of Chinatown and stationed police to keep Chinese inside. When the epidemic spread anyway, federal authorities were called in to help with the containment. They set up roadblocks and inspected railroad passengers at the state line in an attempt to keep the Chinese and "their plague" in San Francisco.

California's governor refused to admit that the plague existed; it would be bad for business. He secured the backing of the state board of health and the Chinese community (which was hiding its sick). San Francisco's newspapers, at the behest of advertisers, ignored proved cases and lampooned city health workers. There was a political stalemate, with the Republican governor on one side and the city's Democratic mayor on the other. Oblivious to human politics and foibles, the plague spread. Finally the Federal government sent in a team of investigators, and in 1901 the governor was forced to capitulate. He stated four conditions for his "cooperation": (1) that the entire operation be kept quiet, (2) that neither the state nor its cities be quarantined, (3) that containment be "pursued with the least possible detriment to our commercial interest," and (4) that the Federal authorities not bill the state for costs.[10]

Thus, in an appropriately disruptive way, _Y. pestis_ completed its world tour. From the steppes of central Asia to China and the Mediterranean, thence to Europe, and finally to the New World was a journey that took over 2000 years. During the passage the bacillus played a role in some of the great changes of history at a cost of untold millions dead along the way.

THE GLOBAL SPREAD OF AIDS

Current evidence indicates that the home base of HIV is central Africa. Understandably, African politicians in 1985–1987 responded to this ascription with counter-charges of "Western imperialistic lying and anti-black racism"; after all, who wants credit for a new pestilence? But this political phase has passed, and there is general agreement on the epidemiological data, which points to central Africa, a region of the tropical rainforest, as the home base of HIV-1 and west Africa as the base of HIV-2.[11]

AIDS was endemic to remote African villages long before it was known or named by Western science. The natives had their own names for it ("the thin sickness") and were familiar with its ravages. In the Ugandan village of Kytera the rate of infection may be as high as 20%, and most of the children are orphans.[12] In 1985 a research team demonstrated that the HIV seroprevalence rate had remained stable since at least 1975 in the village of Yondongi of northwestern Zaire, and this stability might be characteristic of remote rural settings for as long as they remained unaffected by contemporary war and/or commerce.[13] During the 1970s upper-class Zaireans were travelling to European hospitals to get help for a puzzling new "tropical disease." The first authenticated European case from African exposure was the death of Dr. Grethe Rask, who worked at a hospital in Abumombazi in northeastern Zaire near the border with Sudan. Dr. Rask collapsed on Christmas Eve 1976 in Kinshasa, Zaire, and returned to her native Denmark to die in 1977. At that time no one knew what had killed her; now all the symptoms of AIDS are recognizable.

HIV did not stay in the villages. The withdrawal of European colonial power from equatorial Africa, commencing with Ghana's 1957 declaration of independence from Britain followed by Guinea's separation from France in 1958, began a period of war, revolution, and every form of socioeconomic disruption, which continues to the present day. The stability imposed by European powers after they divided up the continent (for themselves) at the Berlin Congress of 1884 dissolved as various African groups vied to seize the reins of power.

The significance of these tumultuous political events for AIDS is that a population that, up to that time, was rural and stable became urban and mobile. People moved and carried their infections with them. For example, Angolan officials estimate that, in the period just before independence from Portugal in 1975, a million people migrated into Zaire. Despite continuing strife in northern Angola, masses of people continue to flow freely back and forth across the border, carrying the virus with them. The highest Angolan seropositive rate is found in precisely those northern border areas. Congo, just north of Angola and sharing a long border with Zaire, has an estimated 10% rate of infection in its urban, sexually active age groups (40% of the continent's population is in this age group). On the other hand, Gabon, the western neighbor of Congo, enjoys a comparatively low infection rate. Apparently it is protected by jungle covering so thick that population movement is impeded.[14] Accurate epidemiological data are hard to gather in Africa, but World Health Organization data indicate that in some major central African cities the seroprevalence rate is many times higher than that in the United States (15.8 per 100,000), and twice the San Francisco rate (110 per 100,000), which is continental America's highest.[15]

The high prevalence rates found throughout central Africa are indirect evidence that the virus has been spreading for some time as a general result of population movement. Equally important is the fact that, unlike in America and Europe, it has been spread largely through vaginal intercourse. Estimates are that three-fourths of the cases result from male/female infection, and the ratio between the sexes is approximately even, as compared with the 12:1 male/female ratio in the industrialized nations. Rapid and disruptive changes in the politico-economic systems have forced men to leave their villages to find work in the cities. There they are separated from both their families and the restraining force of traditional tribal values.

In many cities throughout Africa, Asia, and Latin America, one result of urbanization has been the emergence of a large prostitution industry servicing the sexual needs of this army of displaced men. The shambles of the central African economy are such that the women have no means of support, nothing to sell but their bodies. A century ago this process occurred in America, also as a by-product of industrialization and urbanization, and with a dramatic increase in the rate of syphilis and gonorrhea. Now, however, the disease being spread via the route of prostitution is AIDS. In some places AIDS is known as the "disease of shame," referring to the fact that it is acquired by consorting with or being a prostitute—an African heterosexual stigma, rather than an American homosexual one. Retrospective studies of HIV infection in Nairobi prostitutes indicate that between 1981 and 1985 the rate rose from 8% to 61%. Surveys of the urban prostitute populations of Rwanda, Kenya, and Zaire indicate HIV-1 prevalence rates of 25% to 88%.[16] By comparison, 1988 data indicated that the rate among New York City prostitutes was 12%, and among northern New Jersey prostitutes it was about 49%, while southern Nevada, where prostitution is state regulated, registered the lowest rate.[17]

Other agents strongly implicated in the African spread of HIV are multiple use of unsterile hypodermic needles and a contaminated blood supply. All observers agree that "disposable" needles are simply not thrown away as they should be; the needles are sharpened and reused. This dangerous practice is not the result of ignorance; it is the result of economics. Large city hospitals are underfunded and ill equipped, and rural hospitals are primitive—in neither is anything "disposable." Similarly, even after it became clear in the industrialized nations that the blood supply had to be screened, Africa could not afford the $6 to $8 cost per unit. The United States is spending about $100 million/year to screen the supply to diminish the risk of spreading AIDS through transfusion; that amount exceeds the total public health budget of all the central African nations, which have also to cope with endemic malaria, bilharzia, many enteric ailments, ulcerative venereal diseases, chancroids, and many other diseases.

By whatever mode, the major cities of central Africa became geographic foci of endemicity in the 1960–1980 period, bases from which AIDS could spread to the world. The technology of that spread was air commerce; AIDS is the first airborne epidemic. A traveller could enplane in Kinshasa or Nairobi, arrive in Paris, London, or New York not many hours later, and then, for example, fly on to St. Louis, Missouri, to infect Robert. Actually HIV does not need jet travel. With an incubation period of a decade it is not subject to the time and space limitations that restricted *Y. pestis*, but clearly the airplane made possible HIV's global dispersion in a stupefyingly short period.

Just as it was possible to trace the movement of the bubonic plague from seaport to seaport, it is possible to trace AIDS from airport to airport. For example, AIDS came to Haiti during the late 1960s from two sources: (1) American and European travellers, and (2) Haitians returning home after working in Zaire.[18] Travellers, some infected, arrived by plane. Haiti provided conditions for the spread of AIDS like those of Africa—poverty, poor medical facilities, poor general health, and an exploited, prostituted underclass in which any communicable disease could spread rapidly.

From there, and in sufficient volume to boast epidemic potential, HIV travelled to the United States. First, Haitians escaping the corrupt and brutal Duvalier regime brought AIDS with them to America. However, it is not likely that once they were here, they were important sources of its spread, since they tended to remain in their small, closed refugee communities. Their heterosexual/vaginal infection became an anomaly in the American pattern, which epidemiologists were hard pressed to explain in the early days of the epidemic. The first reports of the CDC simply lumped all Haitians into a high-risk group. The "high risk" designation of an entire nationality was later dropped for political reasons. Second, AIDS was brought back by vacationing Americans. Here the CDC designations did point to an undeniable truth. The accidents of history made the gay community the primary instrument by which the virus was introduced into America in epidemic-level quantities. Haiti was a favored vacation spot for East coast gays. It was exotic, inexpensive, and just a short flight from New York. The HIV that surfaced in New York's gay community in the late 1970s was at least partly a Haitian import.

From New York, Florida, and the Caribbean the virus could spread rapidly to other parts of the nation. But as was the case with the bubonic plague, it did not spread evenly. The plague hit the seaports immediately and then the inland cities that were the most closely connected by commercial ties. In like fashion, the American areas with the highest number of cases are all major hubs of national and international air traffic (the top 10 cities are New York, San Francisco, Los Angeles, Newark, Houston, Chicago,

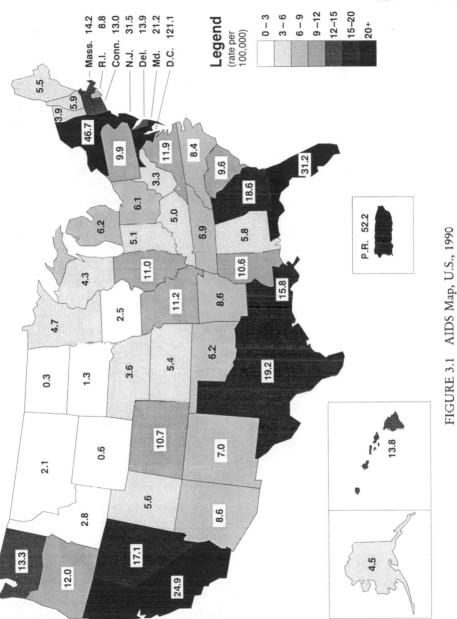

FIGURE 3.1 AIDS Map, U.S., 1990

Source: Centers for Disease Control, "HIV/AIDS Surveillance Report," January 1991, Figure 1, p. 3.

Washington, Miami, Philadelphia, and Atlanta).[19]

The most dramatic example of this process in action comes from the story of the infamous "Patient Zero," Gaetan Dugas.[20] Dugas was an Air Canada flight attendant whose travels during the period 1979–1984 took him frequently to France (the nation most affected by the early spread of AIDS prior to its taking hold in America) and at least 10 American cities; CDC's *Morbidity and Mortality Weekly Report* (June 18, 1982) clearly showed that he was the center of a mini-epidemic, and that fully one-sixth (40) of all reported cases of AIDS up to that time were connected to his coast-to-coast homosexual exploits. No one knows how many others were infected by individuals from this early-infected group. Dugas died, appropriately somehow, while on a flight from Quebec to British Columbia at the age of 32. The infection that he helped spread so widely is still very much alive.

While Dugas was spreading AIDS among homosexuals, Elizabeth Prophet was doing the same among San Francisco's heterosexuals. Ms. Prophet's arrest record for prostitution commenced in 1974 when she was 22. In 1978 her 11-month-old daughter was hospitalized with what we now know was pediatric AIDS; her second (1979) and third children (1982) were also born with AIDS. She died in May 1987 of *Pneumocystis carinii* pneumonia, an opportunistic infection associated with HIV infection. Given present knowledge regarding the course of HIV infection and her personal history, it is likely that she was infected in San Francisco in the mid-1970s. How many men she passed the virus to during her 10-year career can never be known. Two weeks after her death the father of one of her three children also died of AIDS.[21]

Similar stories about the spread of HIV from central Africa could be told about Europe, Asia, the Pacific, and Latin America. The precise epidemiological tracks may never be known as paths cross and backtrack on other paths in this age of rapid mass transit. The detail we have on Patient Zero is exceptional; it is the result of intensive contact tracing in the early days when epidemiologists were trying to establish the nature of the outbreak. But there are other questions that will never be answered. For example, whether Europe was an important staging area for the further spread of AIDS or mostly a recipient is an open question. But there is no doubt that in the 1980s the United States became a most important link in the chain of transport that helped spread AIDS from its original home base in rural, central Africa to over 140 nations and possibly one-tenth of 1% of the world's population in about 30 years.[22] Criticisms of the reluctant and sluggish response of the Reagan administration gain some credence when it is realized that vigorous presidential leadership—the kind elicited by the appearance of Legionnaires' disease, the mistaken fear of swine flu, or the recent San Francisco earthquake—might very well have helped slow and contain what is now a major world epidemic.

THE BUBONIC PLAGUE AND AIDS: A COMPARISON

The bubonic plague and the AIDS epidemic share some features. Each disease was taken from its limited home base and spread throughout the world by the human engines of war and commerce, traveling on the most modern transport of the day. The difference in time that each took to encircle the globe—2000 years and 35 years, respectively—was partly a function of the organisms themselves and partly a reflection of transport technology. Each was and is seen by many people as an act of divine retribution, God's punishment for the various sins of people. And each reactivated ancient prejudices as people sought explanations for their fear and suffering. For the medieval European, the Jew was the answer. The plague came from wells that had been poisoned by Jews and was God's punishment for tolerance of heresy within the Christian community. So Jews were walled up and burned. For the medieval American, homosexuals are the real authors of the epidemic, and everyone is suffering God's wrath for not rooting out this damned minority. In the earlier years of the epidemic there were calls for branding and for rebuilding of the old leprosaria, ghettoes for the sick.

But the similarities stop when the diseases themselves are compared. It is this level of comparison that provokes me to consider the real possibility that AIDS will supplant the Black Death as the archetype epidemic, the new standard for natural catastrophic challenges to the human community.

THE DISEASES

The bubonic plague, in common with most other epidemic-prone afflictions, culled the weak from the population. The old and the young were especially vulnerable, the first to die, the least likely to survive. But AIDS develops primarily in the sexually active age groups that comprise the work force. In Zambia, for example, 68% of the male HIV+ are skilled mineworkers essential to the economy of the nation. In the United States approximately 80% of the 160,000 reported AIDS cases are in the age group 20–49 for both men and women.[23] Compare the U.S., Texas, and San Antonio charts (Figs. 3.2, 3.3, and 3.4). The virus expresses the laws governing its nature regardless of the size or demographic mix of the human group infected. This focusing aspect of AIDS is the source of much popular misunderstanding about the risks of infection. Seroprevalence levels are generally stated as a ratio like 1:100,000 (one case in 100,000 population), but those general population ratio figures do not, in fact, reflect the risks within the population most affected by AIDS. After deducting those over 60 and those under 15, the ratio for the remainder becomes much grimmer.

For example, in Uganda the general rate of infection for the entire population is 1 out of 16; however, if counting is limited to those over 15

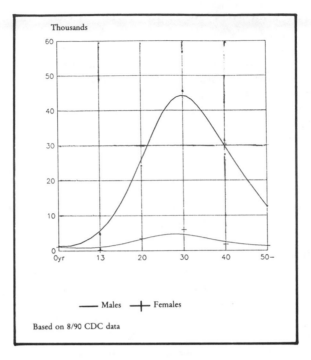

FIGURE 3.2   Age at Diagnosis, U.S. (136,204 cases)

years old, the ratio becomes 1 in 8 infected Ugandans, or 12.5%.[24] It should also be noted that, while it is a disease of sexually active age groups, it is, by the same token, one that targets parents. While it does not directly attack children, it does devastate their lives. In just one area of Uganda, Rakai County, with a population of about 300,000, it is estimated that 40,000 children have lost one or both parents to AIDS.[25] These targeting characteristics become more pronounced as the epidemic takes hold and make AIDS, as compared to the bubonic plague, an infinitely more costly epidemic (see Fig. 3.5).

Another factor to be considered is that the plague had a mortality rate of about 45–50% and the survivors were left with a natural immunity to further visitations. Consequently, like other epidemic-prone pathogens, the plague bacillus gradually killed fewer people as a larger number of resistant adults developed in the population. AIDS, however, attacks the very system that evolved in humans to provide us with immunity to invading organisms; consequently, without effective drugs AIDS is probably 100% fatal. No natural protection can develop except through mutation of the virus itself to

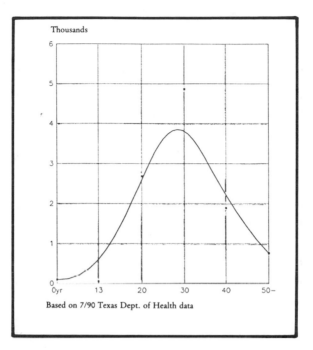

Based on 7/90 Texas Dept. of Health data

FIGURE 3.3   Age at Diagnosis, Texas (10,000 cases)

a less deadly form. In the long term this is likely, since it makes no evolutionary sense for a parasite to kill its host, and most have developed patterns of coexistence. But in the evolution of an organism, the "long term" can be a very long time, especially when one of the measures of time is human death.

SPREADING THE PLAGUE AND AIDS

The pattern of each affliction's transmission and spread is also quite different. An episode of plague was triggered when various factors were coincident. Among many others, these played a part: (1) population densities of specific kinds of rodents and humans, and the relationship of the two densities in a particular site—for example, the crowded living conditions of medieval monasteries made those residing in them especially vulnerable, (2) the construction of human habitation (brick buildings were less prone to rat infestation than others); (3) the extent of population movement between infested areas and other areas; (4) the effectiveness of urban or ocean quarantine systems; (5) finally and importantly, the progress of a particular episode of the plague would itself change the parameters that made it

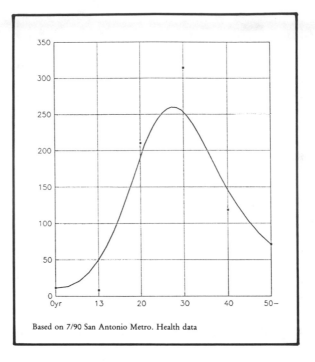

Based on 7/90 San Antonio Metro. Health data

FIGURE 3.4   Age at Diagnosis, San Antonio (732 cases)

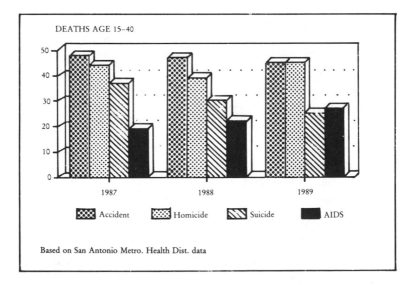

FIGURE 3.5   Males, Cause of Death (San Antonio, 1987–89)

possible in the first place. Thus the plague recurred episodically and unpredictably, like storm waves breaking upon a shore until, eventually, other natural forces exerted themselves to suppress it. The characteristics of the plague, of course, were rooted in the fact that the disease was primarily transmitted from rats through fleas to humans.

On the other hand, AIDS is transmitted entirely within the human community, and generally through some of its most intimate, compelling, and essential behaviors. Unlike the plague, there are no longer any geographic foci of endemicity. AIDS can exist wherever people exist; the human habitat, not some grasslands area, is the natural reservoir. There are no safe areas. Canadian authorities are much concerned about the spread of AIDS among Alaskan Eskimo tribes, which already have a high incidence of venereal disease and whose many languages do not even have an acceptable word for the danger.[26]

Looking back over the decade of tracking HIV from its rural African home base, there appear to be two general patterns of spread. In Africa itself AIDS has overwhelmingly been spread through a combination of (1) vaginal intercourse in an environment with a high incidence of sexually transmitted diseases, (2) an unscreened blood supply, and (3) the use of unsterile hypodermic syringes. Globally speaking, the vast majority of those who have been infected have been infected in these ways. In Europe and America, HIV has been spread largely through anal intercourse, the use of unsterile needles in IV drug use, and vaginal intercourse where one or both partners are IV drug users. In addition, a contaminated blood supply played an early role. Asia still has too few cases to present a pattern, but the widespread use of drugs combined with large and thriving sex industries located in such cities as Bangkok (which has 1500 HIV+ prostitutes and 175,000 IV drug users) will undoubtedly play the central role.[27] The Central and South American scenario echoes that of the United States and Europe, with a contaminated blood supply playing a larger role. It is likely that Latin America is an epidemic disaster area just waiting to be accurately reported.[28] Over the long run, and assuming we do not develop effective strategies for containing AIDS, these differences will even out since HIV has no real preferences; it will spread rapidly or slowly as a function of people's behavior.

However, the sexual transmission of AIDS is the foundation of the exponential (that is, geometric rather than arithmetic) character of its spread. Arithmetic expansion means that A infects B who infects C who infects D; the process is additive. This kind of chain can usually be broken with simple and acceptable measures. Exponential means that A infects B who infects C and D who then infect E, F, G, and H, *ad horrendum*. Dr. Gould of Harvard University reminded his readers of an old children's riddle as a way of visualizing exponential spread. "If you place a penny on square one of a checkerboard and double the number of coins on each subsequent square . . . how big is the stack by the 64th square? The answer: about as high as the universe is wide."[29] Another way to see exponential effect is to take out your pocket calculator and observe how rapidly you go into "overload" when multiplying by the constant 2: $2 \times 2 \times 2 \times 2$. . . . My calculator ran over 1 billion on the 26th pass and gave up. In the American context, exponentiality means that it took 80 months (1981–1982 to January 1988) for the Federal Centers for Disease Control to record the first 50,000 cases; the next 50,000 were recorded in the next 18 months (January 1988 to June 1989); and the third 50,000 is expected by the end of 1990. To put it differently, the first 80 months produced 50,000 cases; the next 36 months added 100,000 more. In the closing months of 1990 new cases were being added at the approximate rate of 2000 per month.[30] The exponential curve will display similar characteristics whether for the nation as a whole or one city within it, such as San Antonio, Texas (see Fig. 3.6 and 3.7).

Theoretically all people-to-people transmissible diseases (like tuberculosis, for example) are spreadable exponentially until such time as they completely destroy the host, but in the real world this does not happen, the stack of pennies falls over, something interrupts the progression. However, sexually transmitted diseases are especially likely to meet the theoretical requirements of exponentiality for the simple reason that we are not, in fact, a monogamous or sexually seasonal species. In Belgium one man infected 11 of the 19 women with whom he had sex over a period from 1983 to 1985.[31] Our religious tradition insists that we ought to be monogamous, but many other traditions disagree, and in any case Christians have seldom practiced what they preached. The divorce and remarriage rate, to say nothing of the existence of abundant extramarital affairs, make clear that we practice serial as well as simultaneous polygamy in both the heterosexual and homosexual world.

These considerations point to one of the most interesting and difficult differences between the bubonic plague and AIDS. Once folk wisdom and science evolved sufficient information about the plague, people could slow transmission and lower risk with relatively commonsense measures requiring no great behavioral changes. In the west Texas pockets of endemicity, people are cautioned not to have any contact with dead rodents and to report their appearance to public health authorities. In the medieval period most people understood that life would be safer in the country, and the rich moved out of the cities if they could. They also understood that population movement had to be curtailed, going so far as to burn at the stake those (poor, not rich folk) who were caught running from an afflicted city and thereby spreading the contagion. Queen Elizabeth I fled the London plague

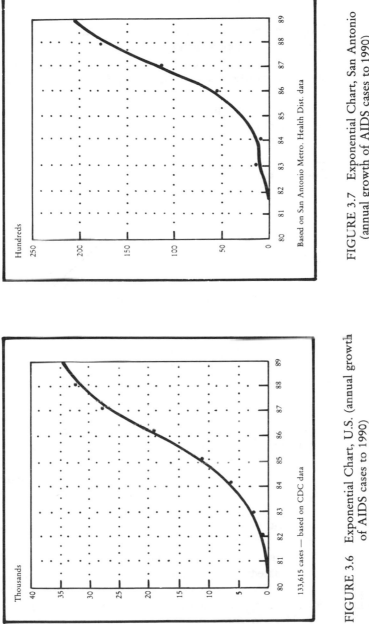

Hundreds

Based on San Antonio Metro. Health Dist. data

FIGURE 3.7 Exponential Chart, San Antonio (annual growth of AIDS cases to 1990)

Thousands

133,615 cases — based on CDC data

FIGURE 3.6 Exponential Chart, U.S. (annual growth of AIDS cases to 1990)

of 1563 to Windsor Castle in the country, and had gallows erected on the access roads to the castle with standing royal orders "to hang all such as should come there from London."

But not picking up a dead rat is not of the same order of magnitude in our behavioral portfolio as not picking up that attractive number at the bar. Clearly a sexually procreated species cannot "just say no" to sex without perishing; we *could* radically change the nature of AIDS spread by somehow separating the infected and uninfected populations, by becoming strictly monogamous, by mating for life, and by always using barrier protection until it was established that both partners were free of the virus.[32] I suspect it will be a cold day in hell before such changes are in effect. Even if we were able to quickly bring about such a striking revolution, the existing world-wide pool would have to be exhausted by death before we could rest easy.

PUBLIC POLICY IMPLICATIONS

The idiosyncratic features of the two diseases have many implications for how we react to them and shape our resulting public policy. I want to mention just a few at this point. The plague was an open, obvious, fast-acting illness. The symptoms were blatant, and when it took hold it moved like wildfire; people died in the streets. It gradually lost its association in the public emotions with outcast groups like the Jews, and more rational methods from public education to rat abatement programs came into use. Of course, it no longer presents an epidemic threat although individual infections do occur. Today the disease responds well to modern antibiotics. History has taught us the hard way that we must move fast, intelligently, and decisively at the first hint of trouble.

AIDS is an altogether different story. Far from being open and obvious, AIDS spread quietly in Africa, Europe, and the United States for decades before alarms sounded. This is one of the qualities of an exponential spread. The virus very slowly establishes a base of one, two, or three cases and then at take-off moves like the Concord, straight up. In 1982 there were only 248 cases reported in the United States; now only nine years later, in January 1991, we have over 160,000 reported cases of AIDS with possibly five times that number of individuals who present some, but not all, of the symptoms required for an AIDS diagnosis.[33] Five years from now epidemiologists project 500,000. Further, in the United States the introduction of HIV was so thoroughly associated with the gay community that decisive political reaction was aborted. As one early commentator put it, "If AIDS had first been imported from Africa into a Park Avenue apartment, we would not have dithered as the exponential march began."[34] That was written in 1987. We still do not have decisive, visible, effective leadership from the White House.

However, the reaction or lack of it both in the United States and elsewhere cannot be blamed solely on such considerations, for it is also true that it is difficult to develop and maintain the necessary sense of public urgency when people are *not* dying in the streets.[35] The great flu epidemic of 1918 flooded hospitals with patients, and on every block someone was sick, relatives were dropping, everybody was at risk and *knew* that they were at risk. My 93-year-old mother-in-law was one of the lucky survivors of both the flu and the 1918 medical treatment for it. HIV, on the other hand, can lie quietly for a decade before showing itself in the form of outward symptoms. Even then, many of the symptoms are ambiguous. Moreover, by that time the patient is frequently bedridden and out of view. Only during late 1986 and 1987 was the public seriously anxious about AIDS, and that was the result of a media blitz on the subject. The blitz was, in turn, tied to circulation, sales, and TV ratings; AIDS was news, just like herpes had been before it. Now, even though the actual epidemic is far more serious, and daily becoming more so, it is just yesterday's news. Out of sight, out of mind. A stupid approach to policy we will all pay for!

Finally, in consideration of the policy impact, as well as my suggestion that AIDS may well supplant the bubonic plague as our archetype epidemic, we have to face the fact that there are no easy and obvious AIDS control programs. A rat abatement program to contain the plague and a "people abatement" program to contain AIDS are very different matters. In the plague of 1664, England's Privy Council joined the two ideas by ordering that houses be boarded up with all residents inside for 40 days, if any resident was reported suffering from plague. Police-state measures such as the quarantines that Cuba has instituted are not available in the democracies unless we want our constitutions to fall victim to AIDS.[36] Those who have proposed major quarantines, branding, imprisonment, health identification cards, mass testing with public lists of the infected, and other draconian measures must consider whether, to paraphrase Abraham Lincoln, our nation can long endure half democratic and half totalitarian.

Notes

1. McNeill, *Plagues and Peoples* (New York: Anchor, 1976), Chap. 5.
2. When epidemics become multinational events they are sometimes called "pandemics" rather than "epidemics." While biologically they are the same events, politically, economically, culturally, and epidemiologically they may be quite different. For example, the epidemiological expression of AIDS in Zaire and the United States is quite different. The male-to-female infected ratio in Zaire is about 1:1, while in the U.S. the great majority of infected are male homosexuals and/or IV drug users. At another level, AIDS will be economically costly to every nation. But it is potentially devastating to Third World economies, while merely burdensome to an economy as powerful as America's.

3. D. Huminer, Rosenfeld, and Pitlik, "AIDS in the Pre-AIDS Era," *Review of Infectious Diseases* 9 (1987): 1102–8. Letter to the editor, *JAMA*, April 21, 1989, p. 2198. Since Robert died of "unknown causes" his blood was stored pending later examination. When that examination was made years later, by scientists at Tulane Medical School, all indications were that he died of AIDS. See R. F. Garry, M. H. Witte, A. A. Gottllieb, *et al.*, "Documentation of an AIDS Virus Infection in the U.S. in 1986," *JAMA* 260 (1988): 2085–87.

4. But see Leigh Page, "Rural AIDS," *American Medical News*, June 3, 1988, p. 3; Randolph Wykoff *et al.*, "Contact Tracing to Identify HIV Infection in a Rural Community," *JAMA*, June 6, 1988, pp. 3563–66.

5. The HIV epidemic may change this classic truth. HIV has heavily infected parts of rural Uganda, Zambia, and Zaire, and Congress has authorized a study in the Ryan White Act of 1990 to track the movement of the virus into rural America. Since people are the carriers, and sex/drugs are the vectors, HIV can go anywhere. If the large numbers still come from the cities, it will simply reflect the fact that that is where the large numbers are, rather than reflect a characteristic of the HIV epidemic.

6. Southwestern Texas had its last outbreak in late 1987–1988. Joe Fohn, "Farm and Ranch Report: Plague Hits West Texas Rodents," *San Antonio Express-News*, February 25, 1988.

7. See Nicola Duplar, "Fleas, the Lethal Leapers," *National Geographic* 173/5 (May 1988).

8. The epidemics that hit the Mediterranean and Europe were not evenly spaced. There was a series that ran from about the time of Christ through the eighth century. Following those there was a long pause until the mid-fourteenth century, when the Black Death inaugurated a new series that continued into the seventeenth century. Finally, a modern series commenced in 1903, starting in India, moving to China, Japan, the Philippines, Hawaii, and, lastly, California and the Southwestern states. This series seems to have burned out in the 1930s, but only after killing some 12 million people.

9. For a very readable account of this fourteenth century plague, complete with contemporary artistic rendering of its devastation, see Charles L. Mee, Jr., "How a Mysterious Disease Laid Low Europe's Masses," *Smithsonian*, February 1990, pp. 67–79.

10. Geddes Smith, *Plague on Us* (New York: Commonwealth Fund, 1941), pp. 323–25.

11. Max Essex and Phillis J. Kanki, "The Origins of the AIDS Virus," *Scientific American*, October 1988, pp. 64–71.

12. Jonathan Mann, James Chin, Peter Piot, and Thomas Quinn, "The International Epidemiology of AIDS," *Scientific American*, October 1988, pp. 82–89. The story on Kytera was filed by Robert Brazell, veteran AIDS reporter. See Lori Heise, "AIDS: New Threat to the Third World," *World Watch* (Jan./Feb. 1988).

13. Nzila Nzilambi *et al.*, "The Prevalence of Infection with Human Immunodeficiency Virus over a 10-year Period in Rural Zaire," *N. Engl. J. Med.*, February 4, 1988, pp. 276–79.

14. See James Brooke, "Virus Discoveries Help an African Outpost of AIDS Research Gain Notice," *New York Times*, February 28, 1988, p. 12.

15. See Federal Centers for Disease Control, *HIV/AIDS Surveillance Report*, September 1990. The highest rate, 48.3 per 100,000, for areas of American jurisdic-

tion are registered in Puerto Rico. Heise, "AIDS: New Threat to the Third World," p. 20.

16. Peter Piot *et al.*, "AIDS: An International Perspective," *Science* 239, no. 4848, p. 574.
17. Bruce Lambert, "Aids in Prostitutes Not as Prevalent as Believed, Studies Find," *New York Times*, September 20, 1988.
18. The Zaire government hired many French-speaking Haitians to fill the posts vacated by departing Belgians.
19. On December 21, 1987, Washington columnist Jack Anderson published a mapping of the United States according to the number of HIV+ per 1000 population levels. Reporters state the map was developed by the Central Intelligence Agency:

2/1000	1.5/1000		1/1000		> 1/1000	
CA	AL	MA	AZ	NM	AK	UT
MD	CO	MI	AR	OK	KY	VT
NV	CT	MO	ID	SD	ME	MN
NJ	FL	NC	IN	WA	WV	MT
NY	GA	PA	IA	WI	WY	ND
DC	HI	RI	KS	MS	OH	OR
	IL	SC	NE	NH		
	LA	TN				
	TX	VA				

The columnist's view of things is fairly well substantiated by current data from the Federal Centers for Disease Control. See the seroprevalence mapping of the nation in U.S. Department of Health and Human Services, Federal Centers for Disease Control, *HIV/AIDS Surveillance* (U.S. AIDS cases reported through January 1990), February 1990, pp. 3, 6–7.
20. Randy Shilts, "Patient Zero: The Man Who Brought AIDS to America," *California Magazine*, October 1987, p. 69.
21. Randy Shilts, "S. F. Hookers Who Made AIDS History," *The San Francisco Chronicle*, August 1987.
22. Dennis L. Breo, "Interview with James Chin, MD: WHO Official Says He Is Still Mobilizing for the Global AIDS Battle," *American Medical News*, November 11, 1988, p. 9.
23. *AIDS Surveillance Report, June 1989*, San Antonio Metropolitan Health District. The national figures are from the bulletins of the U.S. Centers for Disease Control.
24. "AIDS in Africa," *New York Times*, September 19, 1990, p. A10.
25. "In AIDS-stricken Uganda Area the Orphans Struggle to Survive," *New York Times*, June 10, 1990, p. A1.
26. John F. Burns, "Quick Spread of AIDS Seen for Eskimos," *New York Times*, p. 12.
27. Steven Erlanger, "Thriving Sex Industry in Bangkok Is Raising Fears of an AIDS Epidemic," *New York Times*, International, March 30, 1989, p. 3. Lawrence K. Altman, "AIDS Reported Rising in Thai Drug Users," *New York Times*, April 18, 1989. Barbara Crossette, "Bangkok Awakens to the Fears of AIDS," *New*

York Times, November 8, 1987. "AIDS Homes In: Thailand," *The Economist*, February 4, 1989, p. 37. See also the lecture by Dr. Anthony Fauci, Director of the National Institute of Allergy and Infectious Diseases, "Portrait of AIDS in the 1990s," delivered at the Clinical Center of the NIH on December 6, 1989. The lecture is summarized in *Washington HIV News* 1, no. 4 (January 1990) (distributed electronically through the InterUniversity BITNET system).

28. Lindsy Gruson, "AIDS Spreading in Central America," *New York Times*, October 19, 1988.

29. Stephen Jay Gould, "The Terrifying Normalcy of AIDS: The Exponential Spread of AIDS Underscores the Tragedy of Our Delay in Fighting One of Nature's Plagues," *New York Times Magazine*, April 19, 1987.

30. Centers for Disease Control, *HIV/AIDS Surveillance*, from June 1990, Table I, cumulative totals.

31. The case is reported and analyzed by Nathan Clumeck *et al.*, "A Cluster of HIV Infections among Heterosexual People without Apparent Risk Factors," *N. Engl. J. Med.*, November 23, 1989, pp. 1460–62.

32. Review the recommendations in this regard made by William B. Johnston and Kevin R. Hopkins, *The Catastrophe Ahead, AIDS and the Case for a New Public Policy* (New York: Praeger, 1990) (published in cooperation with the Hudson Institute).

33. The distinction between AIDS and ARC has to do with original CDC definitions. AIDS is a strict and elaborate clinical definition (it runs three pages), while ARC (or AIDS-related conditions) is a collection of ailments that in some measure fall short of that definition, although both AIDS and ARC individuals are infected with the virus. The strict CDC AIDS definition makes sense in terms of epidemiological reporting but has been found to be too strict for clinical use. It has had to be considerably modified for use in Africa and other countries, for example. ARC has been largely discarded as a useful category.

34. Gould, "The Terrifying Normalcy of AIDS."

35. See the article by Gina Kolata, "AIDS Advocates Find a Decline in Private Funds," *New York Times*, August 7, 1990, p. A11.

36. Cuba has tested about 80% of the 3.5 million in the sexually active age groups of its population. This has produced 268 HIV+ who are housed in a camp in an isolated part of the island. All Cuban soldiers and citizens who resided in African stations are tested before returning home, and the Cuban government strongly discourages any personal contact between Cubans and the native population. The policy is summed up: "Cubano con cubana." See the story by James Brooke, "AIDS Begins to Spread from War-Riven Angola in Central Africa," *New York Times*, February 19, 1989, p. 4. See "Soviets Introduce World's Toughest Anti-AIDS Measures," *Washington Post*, August 26, 1987.

4

AIDS Research
and Treatment

Back in the spring of 1986 I visited a friend being treated for AIDS at San Antonio's Methodist Hospital. I remember his hospitalization as one long period of uncertainty and pathos. On Monday Teddy would be looking and feeling so well that it seemed likely he would be discharged by Friday. When Friday came, he would be in intensive care, barely breathing. Then, within a week, he was back to a regular room, and back to hope. So it went for almost the whole of his last three months. His care was superb, and the physicians and nurses were obviously skilled and caring. But AIDS treatment was all so new. I can still recall the hushed and worried conferences in the hall as the attending staff asked each other, "What do we do now? What do we do next?"

Things have changed since then, and for the better. I doubt whether the history of medicine presents another example of so much advance in so short a time as there has been in the care of PWAs. Whereas five years ago there was virtually no information, today there are over 120 new journals dedicated to AIDS. There is such an abundance of activity on all fronts that no one can keep abreast of everything that occurs in basic research and treatment. Five years ago receiving a diagnosis of AIDS was tantamount to being sentenced to a rapid and tormented death. Today a multitude of signs indicate that, while there is no cure yet, physicians are developing effective case management techniques. New and more effective treatments are resulting in increased survival time for larger numbers of PWAs as well as an improved quality for the patient's remaining life.[1] An editorial in the *Journal of the American Medical Association* put it this way: "The perception of AIDS as a medical disease is changing. Previously considered fatal in the

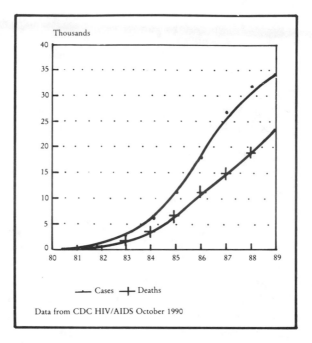

FIGURE 4.1   AIDS Cases and Deaths, U.S. (to 1990)

short term . . . AIDS now is viewed increasingly as a long term disease . . . in which therapy might significantly prolong life and some complications might be totally preventable."[2] The effect of better medical intervention can be seen in a comparison of curves plotting the number of cases and the number of deaths (Fig. 4.1). After 1987 the two curves begin to diverge in a striking fashion, indicating that people are living longer even though the number of infected is increasing. In 1985 about 31% lived longer than two years after diagnosis; by 1987 that figure had reached 49%, and in 1989 approximately 71% were surviving more than two years. PWAs are living longer and, just as important, living better because knowledge is displacing ignorance, and proved technique is replacing trial and error.

However, for the HIV+, the "walking worried," parents, lovers, friends, students, and concerned citizens, there is a down side to the rapidity of development and the flood of coverage. AIDS is a sensational event and gets a sensationalist press; it is often difficult to sort out the wheat from the chaff, the information from the misinformation that bombards our minds. Can you get AIDS from a kiss? Has a cure really been discovered in Kenya? Are drug makers holding back a cure until more get sick, in order to increase sales and profits? And my favorite question: Was the virus transmitted from monkeys to humans through sex in a wild jungle orgy? The obvious tabloid material is easy enough to spot and discount, but there remains the question, Where does one go to get the best information, the most thoroughly examined and documented information, the data which currently is believed valid by responsible people? There is a veritable flood of materials, a flow so vast that specialized journals and newsletters have been developed simply to summarize and disseminate developments.[3] But where can you dip into the torrent?

One important place is *A.T.I.N., AIDS Targeted Information Newsletter, Abstracts and Critical Comments from the Current Literature* (Williams & Wilkins, Baltimore, MD). This monthly newsletter is sponsored by the American Foundation for AIDS Research and is distributed in cooperation with the World Health Organization's Special Program on AIDS. Each month ATIN summarizes articles from over 100 professional journals in molecular biology, virology, immunology, epidemiology, clinical medicine, and treatment, as well as articles germane to the public policy issues raised by the epidemic. It targets a trained and specialized readership, but an occasional perusal can help you get a sense of the complexity and breadth of research taking place. Even if you cannot understand it all, as most assuredly I do not, it can be encouraging to see for yourself how much is going on and how many talented people are dedicated to containing and defeating AIDS. It is also, *sub silentio*, an index to how seriously the scientific community takes the threat of AIDS.

The contents of the May 1988 issue are illustrative and typical of the rich mine of information contained in ATIN. The issue opens with an article summarizing the results of the American Foundation for AIDS Research Forum, which took place in Washington, D.C. on April 9, 1988. This conference brought together some of the nation's leading researchers in a major confrontation and debate on the causes and development of the AIDS syndrome. The forum did not settle all the issues, but it did crystallize the majority and minority positions relating to the causes of AIDS. ATIN then goes on to digest, or give bibliographic notice to, some 318 articles or conference proceedings that had appeared since the previous month. For example, a leading article in the *British Medical Journal* examined the nature and character of heterosexual transmission of AIDS.[4] Another from the *Journal of Infectious Diseases* examined the appearance of cryptococcal meningitis in AIDS patients.[5] An article by a group of immunologists examines the prospects for the development of a vaccine.[6] The examples could go on and on through the 318 references of the May issue. This one issue represents the research of thousands of scientists participating in a global effort not only to isolate causes and develop treatments, but also to confront the nonmedical dimensions of the epidemic. It is an example of the periodicals designed to render AIDS information manageable.

Another approach to fishing for good information would be to read one of the one-volume professional texts that are now available. Any of these works contains everything that the layperson might want to know about AIDS. They are not light reading, but they are worth some effort and, while the nonprofessional will not understand it all, he or she will come away vastly more knowledgeable about what we know and what we do not know about AIDS: (1) Jay A. Levy (ed.), *AIDS, Pathogenesis and Treatment* (New York: Marcel Dekker, 1989); (2) Vincent T. DeVita, Jr., Samuel Hellman, and Steven A. Rosenberg (eds.), *AIDS: Etiology, Diagnosis, Treatment, and Prevention*, 2nd ed. (Philadelphia: J. B. Lippincott, 1988); and (3) Gary P. Wormser, Rosalyn E. Stahl, and Edward J. Bottone (eds.), *AIDS: Acquired Immune Deficiency Syndrome, and Other Manifestation of HIV Infection, Epidemiology, Etiology, Immunology, Control, Treatment and Prevention* (Park Ridge, NJ: Noyes Publications, 1987). Finally, for those with computer modems, these works can be supplemented with a constant flow of current information from one of 19 national and international computer information networks.[7]

If one prefers a less technical approach there are many bulletins designed to convey to PWAs and community care organizations the voluminous information on experimental medical and nonmedical interventions. *AIDS Treatment News*, published biweekly in San Francisco, is an established and reliable newsletter for the nontechnical reader. Its stated purpose is to make a wide range of medical and nonmedical treatment options available in the belief that the survival of PWAs will be enhanced by a combination of individualized therapies.[8] In the July 6 and 20, 1990 issues are summary reports on the many presentations of the Sixth International Conference on AIDS, which met in San Francisco in June 1990. For example, there is information on experiments at the UCLA School of Medicine and Cedars of Lebanon Hospital with injectable Chinese medicines, new data on the use of AZT in combination with other drugs, and disturbing news about the ability of HIV to develop resistance, through rapid mutation, to the drugs used to fight it.[9]

There are many other similar newsletters with varying emphases, as well as occasional bulletins of interest such as Project Inform's *Federally UNapproved Medications for Treatment of AIDS and AIDS Related Conditions: How to Get Them, How to Bring Them Home, and How to Use Them*. Indicating the original "underground" nature (that is, not approved by the pharmaceutical, medical, and/or government establishments) of many AIDS treatments, this bulletin gave its readers advice on how to buy and smuggle drugs available in Mexico.[10] There are also the Gay Men's Health Crisis'

Treatment Issues—The GMHC Newsletter of Experimental AIDS Therapies,[11] the San Francisco AIDS Foundation's *Bulletin of Experimental Treatment for AIDS,*[12] and the *AIDS/HIV Treatment Directory* published by the American Foundation for AIDS Research.[13]

In addition to the information explosion, there has been a weedlike growth of agencies, both private and public, addressing various facets of the epidemic. In the best American tradition, the first on the scene were voluntary, community care groups, privately organized and funded. Most of those operating today were established in the four-year period 1982–1986.[14] As one might expect, the beginning efforts were made in the nation's two most affected cities, with the founding of New York's Gay Men's Health Crisis and the San Francisco AIDS Foundation. Both are now large, successful associations with multimillion-dollar budgets and all the problems typical of middle-aged organizations—complex agendas, internal divisions, and bureaucracies.[15] From this beginning private voluntary organizations (AIDS service organizations or ASOs) spread across the country. There are now over 2500 such groups, supplemented by about 80 organizations representing people with AIDS.[16] In Texas there are 177 private groups; my home city of San Antonio lists 18. I doubt that there is any historic parallel to this explosion of private initiative and organization. The still-to-be-written chapters of this grass-roots response will be among the finest in America's long and proud history of self-help and compassionate care.

On the public side, former Surgeon General Koop issued a call in June 1987 for the creation of a network of care and research agencies to bring some order to the mushrooming agency development stimulated by AIDS.[17] The most important organizational development has been the establishment, under the aegis of the National Institute of Allergy and Infectious Diseases, of a national network of research, training, and evaluation groups concerned with the many faces of AIDS. The components of this network were: intramural AIDS research groups concerned with basic scientific information on the virus; programs designed to attract top scientific minds to AIDS research; AIDS vaccine research and evaluation groups; the National Cooperative Drug Discovery and Development groups; and clinical study groups. Altogether, there are eight specialized levels of federally sponsored and funded groups operating in about 50 cities. These government-sponsored operations are very frequently tied in with university research institutes.[18] Supporting all this with a basic foundation is the HIV Genetic Sequence Database Research Resource of the Los Alamos National Laboratory. And finally, note should be taken of the 13 regional AIDS Education and Training Centers established specifically to provide more and better AIDS care providers.[19]

The metaphor of a flood—even a flash flood—is useful to help visualize the extraordinary activity that AIDS has inspired. It is also useful in another way. A flood probes and exploits with searching, unrelenting fingers every fissure, every indentation, every weakness of the environment. It will find and amplify them all. So it is with AIDS in the scientific-medical sector of America's health care industry. I do not think the epidemic has really created any altogether new professional, organizational, or financial problems, but it has revealed and aggravated those that already existed. This process is very evident when we examine the relations between the main actors in the drama of finding *and* delivering a cure for AIDS.

THE PRINCIPAL WORKERS

Not since the development of the atomic bomb in World War II has there been such a rapid deployment of intellectual and technical energies to focus on one scientific problem. At the Fifth International Conference on AIDS, which met in Montreal, over 5000 papers on various aspects of the diseases were presented; the sixth conference, in San Francisco, heard a like number. That all this effort has not yet borne fruit with truly effective medical routines is mute testimony to the scientific complexity of dealing with viral diseases.

However, there are also nonscientific factors that have negatively influenced the character and speed of our attack on AIDS. Those who are directly involved in fighting the epidemic do not constitute one homogeneous group and do not necessarily share compatible methods or goals. On the contrary, there has been a great deal of disarray among the medical, scientific, and pharmaceutical groups involved. Complicating matters further is an ongoing antagonism between the bureaucracies of the medical, scientific, and pharmaceutical communities, on the one hand, and the nonestablishment ASO groups, on the other. In itself there is nothing unusual in this situation. One of America's strengths is its competitive, pluralistic society, one in which a certain amount of disorganization is normal. However, fighting an epidemic requires speed of action and maximal use of resources. An epidemic is an extraordinary occasion calling for extraordinary and cooperative action. Business as usual prolongs suffering.

Among the professional groups involved in the care and cure of AIDS, the front-line troops are, of course, the clinical physicians engaged in what can only be called a frustrating, no-win trench warfare against the virus. Clinicians are the persons to whom patients look with hope. As a group they are the ones most interested professionally in gaining access to new techniques, drugs, and treatments to alleviate the suffering of the real human beings in their offices. Compared with their laboratory colleagues they are more willing to accept anecdotal or clinical observations that do not meet the strict evidentiary requirements of bench science. They are more willing to try new and unproved approaches, and chafe at the slowness and deliberation of their laboratory colleagues and pharmaceutical and government bureaucracies. As one clinician, Dr. Jay Lalezari, put it, "When you stand at a patient's bedside at two in the morning and he can't breathe because he's suffocating with PCP, you'll try anything."[20] It is this group that most clearly expresses the classical humanitarian, care-giving role of the physician, a role which we mistakenly tend to attribute to all scientists in health care and related fields.[21] Many have actively collaborated, at hazard to their professional careers, in the creation of the large underground network for delivering federally unapproved treatments.[22] It is their clients who are dying right now; and each death is a defeat.

The character of practicing physicians, indeed their very virtues, make it unlikely that a solution to AIDS will emerge from their collective efforts. The clinicians are too much on the front line, too involved with their patients, and too reliant on their own unique, nonreplicable observations emerging from their particular patients (who may or may not be representative of all PWAs). On the other hand, the clinician may become aware of the efficacy of a new treatment (such as aerosol pentamidine for pneumocystis) long before their more cautious laboratory colleagues are willing to "certify" it.[23] Even though multimember clinical practice has now become the industrial norm, individual physicians are still remarkably alone with their patients; one of their greatest needs is some kind of informational network, so that a physician in Kansas City can quickly access the possibly relevant observations of a San Francisco colleague with wider AIDS experience.

In July 1989 Louis W. Sullivan, the Secretary of Health and Human Services, announced the completion of a computerized data base through which AIDS patients and their physicians will be able to get up-to-date information on clinical trials of new drugs and vaccines.[24] This is a major advance in networking, but more is needed. Specifically, what must be developed are some organizational connections that allow separated, individual clinicians, with their wealth of knowledge, to emulate the controlled conditions that ideally prevail in laboratory science. There are a number of important developments and nationally sponsored initiatives in this area, such as (1) the Community Programs for Clinical Research on AIDS, (2) the Clinical Study Groups, (3) the extension of research support to practicing, clinical physicians, and (4) various computer bulletin and networking systems. Most of these are sponsored by the National Institute of Allergy and Infectious Diseases (NIAID) and represent an entirely new thrust in medical research—the attempt to tap into the massive aggregate experience of the front-line physician. Only time will tell how effective these efforts to draw clinicians into the research apparatus of the nation will be.[25]

Laboratory scientists, be they M.D.s or Ph.D.s, the so-called hard scientists, are a different breed. Ordinarily they are removed from the immediate pathos and indignities of death, visiting patients rarely, if at all. Their job is to provide the clinician with the necessary drugs and procedures to prevail. Their primary commitment is not to a particular patient but to a set of protocols called "scientific method" which, if followed rigorously, achieve the closest approximation to objective truth humanly possible. The hard scientist is dedicated to good science not good medicine. Compassion is institutionalized, not particularized; better care-giving is the hoped-for but not the immediately necessary outcome of the work. The personal motivation is not the gratitude of a patient, but the personal satisfaction at having solved a puzzle and discovered new knowledge. The highest accolade for this form of science is the Nobel Prize. This is not to say that the bench scientist is cold, unfeeling, and lacking in human warmth—far from it. We are dependent upon laboratory scientists for those advances in modern medicine that eventually benefit us all. It is just that their priorities, targets, and standards of reference are different, more long range, more targeted to the overall problem than to the specific patient.

Like the clinical physician, the hard scientist can fall victim to his very virtues. He has been the butt of the mad scientist parody in a century of literature (Dr. Frankenstein, Dr. Jekyll), the scientist who has forgotten, in pursuit of knowledge, just who that knowledge is to serve and what limits our common humanity imposes upon research.[26] An example of a genuine dilemma in the AIDS context involves the issue of proper drug-testing protocols. For example, are double-blind, placebo-controlled studies ethically justified in the case of a fatal illness, even though they do provide the most complete evidence of drug effectiveness? In the context of the AIDS epidemic there has been much criticism to the effect that if one is dealing with a doomed patient, then careful and time-consuming adherence to standard protocols for the testing, evaluation, and approval of promising drugs may well be inhumane science—that is, "mad science," perverted hard science.

The literature on AIDS is filled with bitter complaint about the snail-like bureaucratic slowness of the National Institutes of Health, the Federal Drug Administration, and the pharmaceutical industry in releasing new drugs. A recent example involved a panel of AIDS experts convened by NIAID to assess a promising new steroid treatment for *Pneumocystics carinii* pneumonia. PCP is one of the most commonly encountered and serious of the infections associated with AIDS. In May 1990 the panel reached the conclusion that the new treatment was an effective, life-saving therapy. However, it delayed notifying physicians. Bulletins were not issued until October 10, 1990, five months and many respiratory failure deaths later. Even then the notification process was so flawed that many physicians with an AIDS practice did not get the word.[27] On the other hand, there are clear dangers in clinical studies not bound by laboratory controls.[28] At least part of the criticism can be attributed to the fact that the organizations representing the "laboratory perspective" have never addressed the task of educating the public on the need for the 10-year span ordinarily required for the testing and distribution of a new drug.[29] But there is also a point to the argument that an epidemic is no time for business as usual.[30]

People wiser by far than I am have tried to resolve the ethical dilemmas flowing from the clinical and the laboratory perspectives, without notable success.[31] But one thing is clearly true: the longer medical advances stay in the pipeline of review and clearance, the more people will suffer and die. John James, editor of *AIDS Treatment News*, estimated that the cost of delay or failure in the delivery of new, effective treatments at this stage of the epidemic is about 50,000 deaths worldwide every 18 months.[32]

While there are disputable equities and arguments on both sides of the clinical/laboratory debate, there are none that I can fathom in any collision of values between saving lives in an epidemic and making money from an epidemic. It is immoral, basely immoral, to concede priority of claim to the profit motive over that of life itself. Yet there is no question whatever that such moral skewing takes place in the marketplace. Some of our great automakers have knowingly distributed cars that were, to use Ralph Nader's phrase, "unsafe at any speed." Our tobacco industry hawks an addictive carcinogen that has been a subject of condemnation since the time of England's King James I, who wrote a tract on the "stinking weed." Most of our patent medicines at one time were largely alcohol fortified with opium derivatives. And there is no question but that many thousands of hemophilia and surgical patients were infected as a result of the unwillingness of the blood bank industry to incur the additional costs of screening their supply. In the seventeenth century America was founded by merchant-adventurers seeking both material and divine profit. Their entrepreneurial descendants have tended to confuse the two ever since.[33]

The pharmaceutical industry, like all others, is dominated by the profit motive. The skillful caregiving image projected by its advertising tends to obscure the fact that it is an industry that is dedicated to the "bottom line." Like other industries it has its own catalog of disastrous products that were potentially profitable but unsafe, such as thalidomide and the Dalkon shield IUD. One experienced observer of the scene, John James of *AIDS Treatment News*, doubts that, even in the event of a major breakthrough such as the discovery of a "penicillin" for AIDS, the drug would enter the market until time-consuming patent processes had consumed thousands of lives. He cites in this connection the history of a promising drug called Compound Q derived from the root of the Chinese cucumber, *Trichosantes kirilowii*.[34] Laboratory development of the drug in the United States was kept a dark secret for two years. The developers insisted that they wanted to avoid raising false hopes. However, as James pointed out, their concerns on that score dissolved the day their final patent applications were approved and potential profits were protected.[35] Similar stories of profit-motivated delays rather than health-motivated efficiency could be told of fluconazole, aerosol pentamidine, and AL-721.

However, in fairness it should be added that our present patent, liability, and licensing laws offer no incentive to the pharmaceutical industry to make potentially life-saving but still experimental drugs quickly and widely available. As one observer has said, "In the United States today, allowing physicians to use any experimental drug is all cost and no benefit to the company which holds the patent rights."[36] The drug licensing laws under the 1962 Kefauver Amendments to the Food and Drug Act (which were enacted in response to the thalidomide disaster) encourage extreme caution, while the economy offers no money incentive until the number of sick (and therefor potential users) reaches a level where production and distribution is profitable.

The fundamental question acutely raised by the AIDS epidemic is, should we, as a nation, leave control of our national health policy and products in the hands of profit-oriented private associations—be they hospitals, insurance companies, pharmaceutical corporations, or partnerships of physicians in private clinics?[37] If we do, then we support a policy that virtually guarantees either that only the well-to-do will have adequate access to good medicine, or that in order to provide more equal access, private corporations will be given a blank check on the federal treasury through national subsidies. An example of the latter would be the federal funding of AZT (Retrovir). Few individuals could afford the very high price charged (originally about $9,000/year), so Congress allowed the taxpayers to pick up the tab. Burroughs Wellcome Corporation made extraordinary profits, even though the drug was actually developed by the government itself. AZT's profitability is, of course, a corporate secret; however, it has been estimated to be between 900 and 1800%.[38] In November 1990 Congress unanimously amended the 1983 Orphan Drug Act, which had had the unintended effect of making such windfall profits possible. President Bush vetoed the bill, presumably because he believed that such usurious margins of profit were needed and acceptable in order to encourage drug manufacturers to make the medicines we need.[39]

Generally speaking there is nothing wrong with profit, but in the health area it is lamentably easy for profiting to turn into profiteering. For example, it is difficult to understand why pentamidine, when distributed by an

American company to American AIDS patients, should cost from $105 to $300 a vial, while the same drug is distributed in Europe by a French pharmaceutical firm for $30.[40] In the case of AZT it is impossible to understand why a drug developed at taxpayer's expense should be the foundation for private profit. Whatever our answers on these individual cases, there is no question but that AIDS is sharply pointing out that basic reforms and reorganization are badly needed. Prominent medical and business figures are now admitting that our present health care delivery system is slow, chaotic, undependable, overpriced, and economically very discriminatory. In 1989 then Surgeon General Koop said:

> the health care marketplace, although laissez-faire, is not freely competitive and has virtually no moderating controls working on behalf of the patient. So we seem to have a system of health care that is distinguished by a virtual absence of self-regulation on the part of those who provide that care—hospitals and health-care workers, primarily physicians—but distinguished as well by the absence of such natural marketplace controls in regard to price and quality of service.[41]

This is a sad litany for what was once the finest and fairest health care delivery system in the world.

THE PROBLEM OF PROFESSIONAL ETHICS

The epidemic has also revealed an underlying and surprising weakness in the ethical underpinnings of the health care industry. Like most people, I grew up thinking of physicians as motivated by more altruistic standards of service than those that informed other professions. From the early "Dr. Kildare" TV series to current health-care-oriented TV shows, the physician is portrayed as a person striving to be a bit better and a bit more compassionate than most of us. But AIDS has revealed more fear, more prejudice, and more greed than we have wanted to associate with the profession.[42] It has raised anew questions of medical ethics that had long been thought resolved, involving the ethical obligation of the practicing physician to accept risk as an unavoidable accompaniment of his profession.[43] In 1846 the American Medical Association adopted its first code of ethics. It stated clearly: "and when pestilence prevails, it is their duty to face the danger, and to continue their labors for the alleviation of suffering, even at the jeopardy of their own lives."[44] But about 100 years later the age of antibiotics began and we were all, patient and physician alike, lulled into a false sense of security. The grave risks that had always attended the treatment and care of the sick seemed to be reduced to negligible proportions. Among the general population the fear of such diseases as syphilis or gonorrhea receded into the background. The syphilis spirochete that once could destroy the mind and career of Lord

Randolph Churchill now just called for a shot in the rear. The physicians, when they revised their Code of Ethics, left out the pestilence provision. Perhaps it seemed that the entire notion of pestilence was outmoded in the confident new age of antibiotic medicine. AIDS was a rude awakening.

The problem surfaced anew when polls began to show that physicians, nurses, and other health care workers in training were stating that they did not want to care for HIV+ individuals when they entered practice. Other studies suggested that a large number of licensed practitioners were refusing their services on one ground or another. Finally, authentic voices of the profession, such as the *Southern Medical Journal*, were raising questions whether, since seropositivity was "self-inflicted," there should be any ethical obligation to care for AIDS patients. Let the sinners die![45]

Health care workers have argued their right to refuse care on three grounds: (1) that they are facing an unacceptable hazard, (2) that they have a personal need for and right to job satisfaction, and (3) that the care-giving relationship is a free and contractual one. All three sets of arguments have been officially and emphatically rejected by the leading professional organizations. Both the American Medical Association and the American College of Physicians have restated the classical position that "the denial of care to patients for any reason is unethical. . . . Refusal of a physician to care for a specific category of patients—for example, patients who have AIDS or who are HIV+, for any reason is morally and ethically indefensible."[46] This is clear enough and comports with the 1846 Code of Ethics. Further, the American Medical Association now provides an ethics forum in both the journal of the association as well as its newspaper, *American Medical News*.[47] But there can be a great deal of slippage between the official position of any professional association and practice in the field; if you are a patient, it is the attitude of practicing physicians that is crucial, not the policy position of a medico-political elite. Consequently, I think it important to treat the objections to caring for AIDS patients as serious reservations by serious people.

THE HAZARDS OF AIDS CARE

Undeniably there are significant risks involved in caring for AIDS patients, particularly in a surgical, emergency, or intensive-care setting. How great these risks are is extremely difficult, perhaps impossible, to state with any assurance. Research published in the *Journal of the American Medical Association (JAMA)* calculated that the risk to a surgeon of seroconversion was on the order of 1:130,000 to 1:4500. Any estimate with this much spread is at once suspect and certainly not very useful to a person trying to assess his or her occupational risk. What it really says is, "We don't know."[48] On the other hand, merging mathematical models and experience, a San Francisco surgeon with a substantial AIDS clientele calculates that each time he suffers a needlestick injury he has a 1:2000 chance of seroconverting, and since he incurs at least 10 needlesticks per year his yearly seroconversion odds are 1:200. He purchased a large disability policy as a result of his calculations.[49]

A review of the literature on the matter simply underscores the fact that no one has a good grasp on the actual odds. There are too many variables to allow calculations that produce clear, defensible guidelines. Significant variables involve, for example, the kind of service rendered, the condition of the patient, the stage or progress of his infection, the care facilities available and the proficiency of those using them, and the attitudes and training of those rendering care. Only one thing is clear, that the risk is too substantial to be ignored or minimized by official policy statements.[50]

Nonetheless, the simplistic answer seems to be the only one: risk comes with the territory. Admitting that this formula seriously oversimplifies a complex situation involving almost infinite gradations of risk among various types of health care providers, it seems to be the only appropriate place to take a stand on the ethical issues.[51] The annals of medicine are filled with names of those who rendered care at great personal sacrifice and risk. Men like Benjamin Rush, one of the founding fathers of American medicine, cared for yellow fever victims in Philadelphia's 1793 epidemic in the same selfless way many other caregivers have done in countless epidemics down through history. They followed a professional instinct definitively stated by William Boghurst, a London apothecary who lived during the plague of 1666:

> Every man that undertakes to bee of a profession or takes upon him any office must take all parts of it, the good and the evil, the pleasure and the pain, the profit and the inconvenience altogether, and not pick and chuse; for ministers must preach, Captains must fight, Physicians attend upon the Sick.[52]

No one has said it any better; there is little more to say.

JOB SATISFACTION

Another argument supporting the right of the caregiver to withhold service relates to the expectations and satisfaction that motivate the practice of medicine. It is argued that direct service health care providers see themselves primarily as healers whose job it is to get the sick out of bed and back on the job. Consistently failing to do so leads to burnout, loss of morale, lowered efficiency, and professional depression, all to the detriment of their patients. The practice of medicine is already a high-stress occupation without the additional problem of a no-win illness like AIDS. Of course, if a caregiver wishes to undertake this additional stress that is all right, but it ought not to be required ethically or legally.

The sense of professional failure that accompanies the death of a patient is a very real emotion and is not to be treated lightly. No one likes to lose, least of all highly skilled professionals whose self-image and professional reputation are at stake in the mortality rate. The language we use to describe the situation tells how we all feel about it. The doctor "loses" his patient; that is, in a battle of wits with Death, the caregiver has lost. Heroic efforts notwithstanding, Death gets the prize. Incurable AIDS demotes the physician and the supporting personnel from healers to maintenance staff. This is not the satisfying role that a young intern, nurse, or paramedic had in mind to play and, indeed, it must be seriously frustrating and destructive to morale.[53] The problem of burnout in AIDS care is very real and well documented.

This rationale for withholding professional services must be taken seriously and confronted in health care administration. We need to call upon our experience with battlefield medicine to develop programs of support for the caregiver's morale. At the same time, however, it constitutes a reasonable position *only* from those who have already assumed a significant AIDS caseload, *not* from those who anticipate that their morale might suffer if and when they decide to service AIDS patients. The issue is serious, but it is hard to take seriously those in the second group who express it. All caregivers must accept the loss of patients; like risk, this also comes with the territory.

THE DOCTOR-PATIENT "CONTRACT"

By far the most significant and far-reaching argument advanced—the argument most emphatically rejected by the AMA—was that physicians were "just like" the members of any other professional group and should have the right to contract their services for reasons and fees they feel appropriate, as well as to a clientele of their choice. The physician ought to have the legal right to allocate his time and service on the basis of any criteria he thinks applicable, whether they are medical or nonmedical. The architect can decline to design your home, the contractor can refuse to build it, the interior designer can decline to decorate it, and the physician can withhold services to those who live within it. Those who start from this premise insist that there is nothing morally or legally wrong with a caregiver refusing service to an alcoholic, a drug user, a black, a Jew, a homosexual, a communist, or an AIDS victim, not because the caregiver lacks competence (which everyone admits is a compelling reason), but merely because the caregiver dislikes or disapproves of the client as a person.

The first prong of the argument states that physicians are just like other professionals and should be treated as such. But the facts are otherwise. Whether they be Indian shamans, African witch doctors, Mexican *curan-*

deros, or American R.N.s or M.D.s, the populace has always placed caregivers in a special category, and accorded them status, deference, and perquisites commensurate with their importance to society. Caregivers, especially physicians and nurses, are not just plain folk. In contemporary America their professional associations are given quasi-governmental status, with significant regulatory and policing powers. Their importance is signaled by our willingness to heavily subsidize their education in order to guarantee an adequate supply. For example, the individual physician pays dearly in time, dedication, hard work, and money for his or her license; but the truth is that, regardless of whether he or she graduates from a public or a private university, the lion's share of the cost of training the physician is borne by either the taxpayers or private endowments or a combination of both. The cost of a modern medical education is such that, if society were to say, "Pay your own way!" we would have neither doctors nor nurses. By the time practice begins, the American physician is probably the most heavily subsidized product of our graduate education.

No, healers are not ordinary businesspeople. That is their pride, and their burden. Their training is not ordinary, their arts and skills are not ordinary, there is an altruistic and moral aspect to their proper professional motivation, and our reliance upon them is extraordinary. The physicians and their immediate support staffs are special. We think so, and, in truth, so do they. Many of their professional associations are currently arguing before state legislatures in support of special limits on malpractice liability, and their arguments always commence with the assertion that their services are essential to society. Health caregivers demand, deserve, and receive a special place in our social economy; I would argue that, as a consequence, society has the right to place them under obligations not shared by other professionals and, at minimum, insist that they stand fast and do their job in a time of epidemic.

The second prong of the argument asserting that caregivers should have the same liberty of contract to grant or withhold services as other professionals is superficially appealing. It does tie in with the powerful American tradition of free enterprise capitalism, which insists that state restraint on liberty of contract needs strong and special justification. However, in the face of this basic tenet of our national political faith, various groups have successfully argued a compelling case in many areas. Statutory and case law expressions of policy are sharply limiting individual contractual choice for the greater good of society. Within the past 50 years the U.S. Supreme Court and the Congress have ruled that services in the following areas may not ordinarily be granted or withheld on the basis of racial, ethnic, or gender considerations: education; employment; public facilities, from buses and planes to golf courses; private facilities, like restaurants, motels, hotels, or theaters, which cater to the public; rentals or sales of homes by owners or realtors; and admission to private, but business-oriented clubs. It takes no great leap of imagination to frame an argument, if one is really needed, that health care must not be denied to the sick, regardless of who the sick are. I can think of no better way for the caregiving profession to encourage the development of a completely nationalized system than to insist on a contractual right of discrimination when the political and legal trends are clearly in the opposite direction.

It is unlikely, however, that constitutional and/or occupational scruples motivate the objections to treating HIV+ individuals. Much more likely is an understandable but unacceptable fear, and completely intolerable bigotry.[54] Church-defined and -transmitted hatred of homosexuals, and a cultural disdain and fear of IV drug users (especially black and Hispanic ones) are the headwaters of much policy and behavior in America's reaction to this epidemic. The patent fact that the groups earliest affected in the United States were male homosexuals and IV drug users allowed underlying hatreds to surface in many forms, including that of withholding health care.[55]

No caregiver has suggested that for reasons of occupational safety, job satisfaction, or constitutional law, pediatric cases be left untreated and that children be refused care. On the contrary, the care of pediatric AIDS victims is well funded and staffed. Children are the "innocent victims"! The rest are sinners and deserve to die. No more than 13% of the federal health budgets prior to 1990, which ran into the billions, were earmarked for direct care for teens and adults. The Ryan White Act of September 1990 hopefully may change that (see Chapter 6).

History offers many examples of caregivers refusing or corrupting their services for ideological, political, religious, or other personal, nonmedical reasons, but none seem to offer much support in the current American context. Nazi physicians refused treatment to Jews, Southern whites turned away blacks, and Soviet psychiatrists have placed themselves at the service of state security by certifying political dissidents as insane. However, no one suggests that these are models that should be emulated in America. The Jews, the blacks, and the dissidents had one thing in common: they were outcasts in their own societies, just as the homosexual and the IV drug user are today.

Over 600 years ago a surgeon advised his students, "If you are asked to treat a patient with no chance of recovery [because of infection with bubonic plague], say that you will be leaving town."[56] It seems at times that we have progressed too little a distance. There are 600,000 physicians and 180,000 dentists in the United States, but a shortage of those who will take AIDS cases. Five percent of the nation's hospitals care for one-half the cases.

Private physicians are not counseling their patients on AIDS, and Surgeon General Antonia Novello's call for help goes unheeded.[57] Altogether too many of our doctors and dentists have left or are "leaving town" to escape the political and personal impact of the AIDS epidemic.

NON-MEDICAL THERAPY

There is an old saying that fits the situation in AIDS perfectly: "When there is no cure, there will be a Thousand Remedies." The failure thus far of science to develop a cure or effective long-term management has led to a proliferation of therapies that hold out the promise of accomplishing what mainline medicine so far cannot. Perusing *Healing AIDS*, a monthly periodical devoted to "alternative" approaches,[58] reveals a rich array of methods including homeopathy; chiropractic; massage; acupuncture/acupressure; Chinese herbal medicine; psychoimmunity; vegetarianism; macrobiotics; spiritualist channeling; crystal healing; art and music therapy; "energetics"; various body "detoxification" regimes; diets using garlic, blue-green algae, Echinacea, shitake mushrooms, or wheat grass; and many forms of yoga, stress reduction, breath control, meditation, or "positive thinking or visualizing," including the currently popular *Course in Miracles*[59] or Louise Hay's *You Can Heal Your Life*.[60]

There is little new in all this. Dietary, pseudo-scientific, and mystical modes of healing, such as laying on of hands, are as old as sickness. Various forms of faith healing are prominent features of America's fundamentalist, born-again evangelical, and New Age movements. Homeopathy is almost 200 years old and was widespread in nineteenth century rural America. Some forms of traditional Chinese medicine express a thousand years of experience. Yoga's ability to achieve stress reduction and body control have been refined over centuries. The ancient Romans believed strongly in the curative properties of certain crystals and gemstones. Europeans and Americans have long enjoyed "detoxifying" their bodies with mud baths and sulfur springs at "curative" spas. Since the mid-nineteenth century cereal and graham cracker craze, Americans have taken up one "health food" or dietary enthusiasm after another. The use of certain vegetables and/or herbs is also ancient. In 1664 the London College of Physicians recommended the following for those afflicted by the plague: "[T]ake a great onion, hollow it, put into it a fig, rue cut small, and a dram of Venice treacle; put it close stopt in a wet paper, and roast it in the embers; then apply it to the tumor." In addition, fat people were advised to stay out of the sun, and garlic was to be eaten raw as well as kept in one's shoes.[61]

The alternative approaches have some conceptual elements in common, even if their particular methods vary greatly. Generally they reject conventional Western medicine's overwhelming reliance on the germ theory of illness, that is, the position that our illnesses are usually traceable to an invading bacterium, fungus, or, as in the case of AIDS, virus. For example, chiropractic is notable in its rejection of germ theory. The alternative approaches tend to stress the mind/body connection, and the influence of the mental or spiritual state upon the body's well-being. For Christian Scientists this connection is all-important; physical illness is conceptualized as a delusion, the product of a spiritually imperfect mind. Finally, there is much common agreement that effective treatment must be holistic; it must deal with the whole person, not just an affected limb or an invading bacterium.

It is undeniable that faith and will power can heal some maladies, can make even more at least tolerable, and finally can help in the treatment of all of them. Any physician can attest to the importance of the patient's mental and emotional outlook. Insofar as these various approaches and their remedies serve as a means of triggering the curative powers of mind, there can be no objection to them. However, the alternative therapies share a common difficulty in establishing any demonstrable, replicable connection between their remedies and the patient's recovery. Furthermore, they lack the standardized educational training and requirements characteristic of established medicine. Because of these factors, they have an unsolvable problem in defining the fake healer, the fraud, the incompetent. While there are criminals and charlatans in both conventional and non-conventional healing, the varied alternative therapies have meager means of policing their fields. Thus alternative healing is exceptionally vulnerable to the intrusion of the fake healer, the medical con man, the seller of "snake oil" for whatever ails you, including AIDS. As far as I know, no alternative therapy sponsors a national hotline (1-800-776-CERT), such as is provided by the American Board of Medical Specialties, through which the consumer can check on the training and credentials of a physician before employing him or her as a healer.[62]

It is unfortunately true that wherever there is sickness and suffering, a certain vulture-like subgroup of our species will descend from the skies to feed. A number of borderline fraudulent charities have been established to solicit funds (usually for the already well-funded, but emotionally appealing children's cases). Generally they donate 10% of the take to AIDS care, and keep the rest for "administrative expenses." Before donating any substantial amount, it is always wise to check with your community's AIDS service organization. Furthermore, many devices already familiar to fraud investigators have reappeared, retrofitted for AIDS, from simple magnetized bracelets to "draw out the virus," to elaborate and costly machines that have no effect other than enriching the seller. My favorite is a hi-tech application of eighteenth- and nineteenth-century phrenology, the "science" (favored by barbers) that asserted that one could diagnose and treat ailments by reading the forms and indentations of the human skull. The contemporary machine adaptation resembles a Star Trek helmet of clear plastic fitted with a large number of sliding needlelike probes. These probes (replacing the old phrenologist's fingers) are fitted to the skull and, through electronic circuitry, "read" a diagnosis. Then, with a mere flip of the switch, imaginatively named electric charges are directed to the appropriate portions of the head to effect a "treatment."[63] It is easy to laugh at this stuff—until you are dying, that is.

What has happened in recent years is that all of the fakes have turned from the thoroughly plowed fields of cancer and rheumatoid arthritis to AIDS. Some of the so-called medications can do great damage; for example, "hyper-oxygenation" treatment using 35% concentrations of hydrogen peroxide is responsible for one death and four hospitalizations in Texas. However, this has not stopped a young friend of mine from trying it. Moreover, false therapies can promote delay in implementing the effective medical treatments now available, like low-dose AZT or pentamidine.

Given all the reservations, however, the fact remains that those offering alternative therapies, both the honest and the dishonest, will continue to flourish as long as conventional medicine falls short.[64] Whatever can be said about the efficacy of their remedies, they do offer hope and, with or without AIDS, a world without hope is a dismal place to be.

Notes

1. Largely as a result of AZT and pentamidine, the survival prospects have increased from about nine months (after diagnosis) to nearly two years. See, for example, Editorial *JAMA*, November 25, 1988; Centers for Disease Control, *Draft Proposals for Early Intervention*, Fifth International Conference on AIDS, Montreal, Canada, June 1989; A. E. Glatt *et al.*, "Treatment of Infections Associated with Human Immunodeficiency Virus," *Medical Intelligence*, 318, no. 2, May 1989, pp. 1349–1448. Probably the most dramatic therapeutic improvement has been the use of aerosol pentamidine as a prophylactic against *pneumocysistis carinii*, which in the early years of the epidemic (and still in the Third World) was the most deadly and common form of opportunistic infection. Also see Roger Rickleps, "Thanks to New Drugs, Patients Are Surviving and Working Longer," *New York Times*, September 2, 1988, p. 1.
2. "Editorial: Improving Survival in Acquired Immunodeficiency Syndrome: Is Experience Everything?" *JAMA*, May 26, 1989, p. 3016. Also see "Editorial: The Rocky Road to Effective Treatment of Human Immunodeficiency Virus (HIV) Infection," *Annals of Internal Medicine* 110, no. 1, (1989): 1; "Editorial: Controlled Trial Methodology and Progress in Treatment of the Acquired Immunodeficiency Syndrome (AIDS)," *Annals of Internal Medicine* 110, no. 6, (1989): 417.
3. Stephen A. Berger, an Israeli physician at Tel-Aviv Medical Center, with tongue in cheek, calculated that, given the rate of increase in AIDS articles between 1982

and 1986, by the year 2263 the AIDS category of the *Index Medicus* (an international index of all medical articles) would require a volume all by itself to index a projected 1,036,348 reports for that year. See *N. Engl. J. Med.*, December 3, 1987, p. 1479.

4. A. M. Johnson, "Heterosexual Transmission of Human Immunodeficiency Virus," *British Medical Journal*, April 9, 1988, p. 1017.

5. W. E. Dismukes, "Cryptococcal Meningitis in Patients with AIDS," *Journal of Infectious Diseases* 157, no. 4 (April 1988): 624.

6. T. J. Mathews, Lyerly, Weinhold, Lanlois, Putney, and Bolognesi (Duke University Medical Center), "Prospects for Development of a Vaccine against HIV-Related Disorders," *Clinical and Immunological Newsletter* 8, no. 4 (April 1987).

7. Lois Levine, "AIDS Online," *AIDS Patient News* 1, no. 1, January 1988, p. 17. Other interesting and useful publications are: *CDC AIDS Weekly*, (Charles Henderson Publications, Atlanta, GA). The title suggests that this is sponsored by the U.S. Centers for Disease Control, but it is actually privately published. Another is *AIDS Clinical Digest*, (American Health Consultants, Atlanta, GA). For electronic databases, networks, etc., see the summary of existing services in *CDC AIDS Weekly*, October 17, 1988, p. 6.

8. John S. James (ed.), *AIDS Treatment News* (P.O. Box 411256, San Francisco, CA 94141).

9. See *AIDS Treatment News* July 6 and 20, 1990. The New York Gay Men's Health Crisis Center, *Treatment Issues, the Center Newsletter of Experimental AIDS Therapies*, February 8, 1988.

10. Project Inform, 25 Taylor St., Suite 618, San Francisco, CA 94102.

11. Write to Gay Men's Health Crisis, Department of Medical Information, 129 W. 20th St., New York, NY 10011, for information.

12. San Francisco AIDS Foundation. Call 415-863-2437 for information.

13. Call 212-719-0033 for information.

14. National Directory. See note 16.

15. For a highly personal history of the New York group see Larry Kramer, *Reports from the Holocaust: The Making of an AIDS Activist* (New York: St. Martin's Press, 1989). Kramer, an author and playwright, was one of the founders of the Gay Men's Health Crisis. But the organization quickly became too "establishment" for his tastes, and he became a vocal opponent and gadfly. He later organized ACT UP, a confrontational advocacy group. Both are active groups.

16. For a complete listing see The U.S. Conference of Mayors, *Local AIDS Services, The National Directory January 1990* (available for $15 from the Conference of Mayors, 1620 Eye St. NW, Washington, D.C. 20008). For a study of the upstate New York experience see Donald B. Rosenthal, *The Institutionalization of AIDS Service Organization: The Upstate New York Experience*, paper prepared for delivery at the 1989 Annual Meeting of the American Political Science Association, Atlanta. Dr. Rosenthal is at the State University of New York at Buffalo.

17. C. Everett Koop, "An AIDS Care Network—the Time Is Now," *AIDS Patient News* 1, no. 1 (June 1987).

18. For a summary, complete with locations and supervising research personnel, see National Institute of Allergy and Infectious Diseases, *Dateline: NIAID, AIDS Research Issue* (Washington, DC: National Institutes of Health, November 1987).

19. "Feds Triple AIDS Training for MD's," *Medical World News*, February 8, 1988, p. 59.

20. Quoted in "Advance in AIDS Treatment," *New York Times*, November 14, 1990, p. A1.

21. See the moving portrayal of a young physician and the impact of AIDS care on his maturation as a doctor in William A. Check, "Growing Up Fast: A New Generation of AIDS Physicians," *Observer* (American College of Physicians) 9, no. 10 (November 1989): 1.

22. See the story of Dr. Stephen Herman, Director of Research at Stephens Pharmaceuticals, in Joyce Niles, "AIDS Researcher Arrested," *Internal Medicine World Report*, March 1, 1990, p. 12.

23. A current example of experimental treatments being tried is hyperthermia (extra-body heating of the blood) used on a Kaposi's sarcoma patient. Dr. William D. Logan and Dr. Kenneth Alonso, Foundation for Virology and Oncology, reported impressive results in inhibiting HIV replication in a press release of May 31, 1990, issued at Atlanta Hospital. However, a team of reviewers from the National Institutes of Health found no merit in the treatment and did not recommend that it be continued. Dr. Alonso's last treatments were reported from Mexico City.

24. *Health InfoCom Network News* 2, no. 31 (1989): 16 (distributed electronically on the InterUniversity BITNET system), news release date, July 18; issue date, August 28. The network is called The AIDS Clinical Trial Information Service.

25. See the announcement of Anthony Fauci, MD, Director of NIAID, and the accompanying article in *American Medical News*, December 9, 1988, p. 3. There is a good discussion in *AIDS Treatment News*, nos. 84 and 85, August 1989.

26. In this connection it is worth noting that every university in the United States must have a special committee to review all research proposals that involve humans. This is to guarantee that humans not be used inhumanely.

27. Gina Kolata, "News of Advance in AIDS Treatment Delayed 5 Months," *New York Times*, November 14, 1990, p. A1. See also the follow-up response from NIAID in the *New York Times*, November 16, 1990, p. A13, and the analysis in *AIDS Treatment Issues, The GMHC Newsletter of Experimental AIDS Therapies*, vol. 4, no. 8, p. 3, November 30, 1990. The charges and responses are well summarized in *Internal Medicine World Report*, December 1990, p. 4, and January 15, 1990.

28. A case in point was the controversy that developed around unorthodox, semi-underground clinical "tests" in 1989 of Compound Q, a promising antiviral drug. See Gina Kolata, "Critics Fault Secret Effort to Test Aids Drug," *New York Times*, September 17, 1989, p. 21, and *New York Times*, September 20, 1989, p. 10.

29. The standard drug development and approval process breaks down approximately like this:

    Preclinical testing (years 1 & 2): The phase during which the safety and biological activity of the new drug is tested, frequently on animals.

    Phase I testing: Testing to determine safety, dosage, toxicity on humans using small groups of *healthy* volunteers (under 100). Seventy percent of the Investigational New Drugs (INDs) will pass this stage.

    Phase II testing (years 4 & 5): The drug is tested on 100 to 300 *patient* volunteers to evaluate effectiveness, possibly dangerous side effects, and so on. Thirty-three percent of INDs will pass this stage.

Phase III testing: Tests on 1000 to 3000 *patient* volunteers to verify Phase II and monitor for long-term effects. Under new "expedited review" procedures these two phases can be combined to shorten the approval process for new medicines addressing life-threatening diseases like AIDS. Twenty-seven percent of INDs will pass Phase III.

Food and Drug Administration Approval (years 9–11): This phase involves FDA review of all the documentation (test results, lab findings) that accumulate. About 20% of all INDs will survive the process and gain FDA approval.

After approval there is still elaborate safety monitoring as the drug goes into manufacturing, distribution, and use.

30. See the interesting discussion of the problem by John S. James, "The Drug Treatment Debacle, Parts 1 & 2," *AIDS Treatment News*, nos. 77–78, 81–82 (1989).

31. A good brief introduction to the problem of differing perspectives was written by Natalie Angier, "Cultures in Conflict: M.D.'s and Ph.D.'s," *New York Times*, April 24, 1990, p. B5.

32. John James, *AIDS Treatment News*, no. 77, p. 4. James points out that in an exponential progression, such as applies roughly to this epidemic, the last doubling of case numbers before a medical advance or cure is found will account for about one-half of the cumulative total of AIDS deaths throughout the entire epidemic.

33. In the 1830s Alexis de Tocqueville observed that the single-minded drive for profit was one of the characteristics that set apart the American from other cultures of the West. See his classic, *Democracy in America*, vol. 2 (Phillips Bradley, ed.) (New York: Knopf, 1945), pp. 247–248.

34. See *New York Times*, Medical Sciences Section, April 18, 1989; *Business Week*, April 24, 1989; *AIDS Treatment News*, April 21, 1989.

35. *AIDS Treatment News*, April 21, 1989, p. 5.

36. John S. James, "Needed: Compulsory Licensing of Pharmaceuticals?" *AIDS Treatment News*, May 19, 1989, p. 4.

37. As an example of the problems see "Correspondence: The Pressure to Keep Prices High at a Walk-in Clinic," *N. Engl. J. Med.*, January 19, 1989, p. 183.

38. "AIDS, Drugs, Need and Greed" (editorial), *New York Times*, September 29, 1989, p. 24. *Australian AIDS News* (distributed electronically on the Inter-University BITNET system), October 28, 1989, reported a major debate in that country about the importation of AZT as a result of such reported profits.

39. *San Antonio Express-News*, November 10, 1990, p. 4G.

40. Gina Kolata, "AIDS Group Plans to Buy Drug for Less in Europe," *New York Times*, September 25, 1989, p. 11. The American manufacturer is Lyphomed of Rosemont, IL. The firm was granted "orphan status" for its product by the Federal Food and Drug Administration, even though the drug is not even patented. "Orphan status" means that the firm has a seven-year legal monopoly on manufacture and distribution, protected by Federal law. There is no market competition restraining the price. Therefore Lyphomed charges whatever the traffic will bear. The same is true of Burroughs Wellcome's AZT.

41. C. Everett Koop, "The Health Care Mess," *Newsweek*, August 28, 1989, p. 10. See also *San Antonio Express-News* coverage of a San Antonio address given by Koop on June 4, 1989.

42. For various analyses see David E. Rogers and Eli Ginzberg (eds.), *Public and*

Professional Attitudes Toward AIDS Patients, A National Dilemma, Cornell University Medical College Fifth Conference on Health Policy (San Francisco: Westview Press, 1989); and Christine Pierce and Donald Van DeVeer (eds.), *AIDS, Ethics and Public Policy* (New York: Wadsworth, 1988).

43. There is a good summary of the arguments in *N. Engl. J. Med.*, 321, no. 19, (1990), pp. 1334–36.
44. As quoted in A. Zuger and H. M. Stevens, "Physicians, AIDS, and Occupational Risk, Historic Traditions and Ethical Obligations," *JAMA*, October 9, 1987, p. 1926.
45. See, for example, Richard Goldstein, "AIDS and the Social Contract," *The Weekly Newspaper of New York*, December 29, 1987.
46. Statement adopted by the ACP in 1987. See *New York Times*, March 13, 1987, p. A21; July 10, 1987, p. D18, and November 13, 1987, p. A14 for reactions and official statements of the medical associations. And see the *Interim Report on the Prevention and Control of AIDS* adopted by the AMA's House of Delegates at the 1987 Annual Meeting at Chicago, June 21–25, 1987.
47. *American Medical News*, February 16, 1990, p. 49, for the current position of the AMA and its new programs.
48. M. O. Hagen, *et al.*, "HIV Occupational Risk," *JAMA* 259 (1988): 1375. And see M. Brown, *et al.*, "The Third International Conference on AIDS: Risk of AIDS in Healthcare Workers," *Nursing Management*, March 1988, pp. 33–36.
49. Sari Staver, "One in 250 HIV-Infected Sticks Transmits Virus—Studies," *American Medical News*, January 13, 1989, pp. 3, 19.
50. See "Commentary: Why Fear Persists: Health Care Professionals and AIDS," *JAMA*, December 16, 1988, p. 3481; Theodore Hammett and Walter Bond, "Risk of Infection with the AIDS Virus Through Exposures to Blood," *AIDS Bulletin* (U.S. Department of Justice, National Institute of Justice), October 1987; Richard Ratzan and Henry Schneiderman, "AIDS, Autopsies, and Abandonment," *JAMA*, December 16, 1988, p. 3466.
51. See the special report, "Fearful Healers," *New York Times*, November 11, 1990, p. A1.
52. Quoted in Zuger and Stevens, "Physicians, AIDS, and Occupational Risk." This is an excellent preliminary exploration of the subject.
53. See the interesting commentary, "Supporting the Health Care Team in Caring for Patients with AIDS," *JAMA*, February 3, 1989, p. 747.
54. See the analysis of Dr. Molly Cook, "HIV Fear Tied to Homophobia and Racial Bias," *Internal Medicine News*, February 15–28, 1990, p. 1 *et seq.*
55. One of the many ironies of the epidemic's course in America is that the homophobia that underlies the denial of care is easily traceable to the "Judeo" part of the Judeo-Christian tradition and the Pauline theological foundation. But the same Jewish culture has produced a firm legal and ethical mandate commanding physicians to heal all patients without regard to their age, sex, race, creed, disease, or lifestyle. See "Jewish Law and the Obligation of the Physician to Heal Patients with AIDS," *JAMA*, April 21, 1989, p. 2199.
56. Quoted in Zuger and Stevens, p. 1925.
57. Bruce Lambert, "AIDS War Shunned by Many Doctors," *New York Times*, April 23, 1990, p. A1.
58. *Healing AIDS, A Magazine of Healing Tools, Resources and Aids* (3835 20th St., San Francisco, CA 94114).
59. Published by The Foundation for Inner Peace (Tiburon, CA, n.d.).

60. Louise Hay, *You Can Heal Your Life* (Santa Monica, CA: Hay House, n.d.).
61. AIDS patients are also advised to stay out of the sun or use a high-protection sun block. It has been demonstrated that ultraviolet radiation has a significant impact on activating HIV. And one of the nation's longest surviving PWAs (now dead) credited his longevity to a daily diet of raw garlic.
62. The hotline is published in 2000 Yellow Pages directories, and can access information on about two-thirds of the nation's 800,000 physicians who have ABMS board certification in some specialty.
63. See *American Medical News*, April 1, 1988.
64. A 1989 survey showed that one-fourth of all patients were trying treatments that had neither the approval of the FDA nor that of their physician. These included megadose vitamins, fetal sheep blood injections, and unapproved drugs. *American Medical News*, December 22–29, 1989, p. 21.

5

Avoiding AIDS:
The Problem of Behavior

We live surrounded by risk that, for the sake of our emotional balance, we ignore as much as possible. The law requires us to strap on seat belts in an effort to cut the more than 50,000 highway deaths per year. Former Surgeon General Koop's number one priority was not AIDS, but the elimination of smoking, which is implicated each year in over 150,000 deaths—three times the number killed in the Vietnam War. Swimming, motorcycles, electrical, and handgun accidents account for another 40,000. Truly, living is dangerous to your health. Torts, a major field of the law, flowers in the dangerous but beautiful garden of our collective lives. A major risk of living has always been that of encountering in some fashion or the other one of the organisms that prey upon us, be it a shark or a bacterium. HIV has added another danger to an already long list. Accompanying every form of risk there are avoidance possibilities which flow from the nature of the predator itself. Thus it is unlikely that a shark will bite you on land, although any ocean fisherman can tell that it can and has happened. Similarly, risk of infection with HIV can be diminished to tolerable levels by simply showing proper respect for the modes of transmission by which the virus is transferred from one host to another.

As an introduction to the topic of avoiding AIDS, here is an approximate rank ordering of risk activities, as I read the data. The intervals between each category are not equal. The rank ordering from greatest to least is based upon the possibility that you will be infected if you are involved, willingly or otherwise, in this activity, and there is HIV contamination:[1]

1. Transfusion of HIV-contaminated blood or blood products—the direct introduction of the virus into the bloodstream.

2. The use of shared, unsterile apparatus for injecting drugs, in or out of health care settings.
3. Being the recipient partner in anal intercourse during which no condom is used.
4. Industrial-medical negligence and/or accident.
5. Being the recipient partner in vaginal intercourse during which no condom is used.
6. Being the insertive partner in vaginal intercourse during which no condom is used.
7. Being the insertive partner in anal intercourse, during which no condom is used.
8. Oral sex (receptive fellatio).
9. Anal intercourse with condom protection.
10. Vaginal intercourse with condom protection.
11. Transfusion of screened blood or blood products.

Other than being born to an infected mother (25% chance of transmission) there are NO other known possibilities than the above and their variations.[2] A recent survey of 14 separate American and African studies seeking to document various modes of transmission concluded that there was no credible evidence of seroconversion other than through the above routes.[3] There are no documented instances of seroconversion due to human or insect bites; sitting on toilet seats; donating blood; sharing foods, glasses, straws, or cooking and eating utensils; shaking hands; or hugging. There are no documented cases of seroconversion as a result of exposure to infected individuals in the occupational pursuits of firefighting, law enforcement, emergency response technicians, or general office or educational work. In short, AIDS is not easy to get and/or transmit; if it were, the world would be in much bigger trouble.

However, there are innumerable variations on the risky behaviors that create nuances that, in real life, affect the relative placement of risk. For example, the insertive partner's risk (nos. 6 and 7) is seriously heightened if he is uncircumcised or has genital ulcers.[4] Similarly, it makes a huge difference if an IV drug user patronizes a "shooting gallery" or uses his own "works" at home. Further, it is impossible to disentangle some behaviors, like kissing and intercourse, so that attribution of seroconversion to intercourse alone is certain. The difficulties in getting precise statements in this entire area are reflections of three factors: (1) the paucity of data on sexual behavior in general; (2) the newness of the entire field of retroviral research; and (3) the highly conditional nature of statistical statements.

LIES, DAMNED LIES, AND STATISTICS

AIDS has not made dangerous behavior that was all that safe before. But it does force us to reassess risk and adjust our attitudes and behavior. We need to think about how to evaluate, in personal terms, the various statements that bombard us daily. For example, people read in the newspapers that the chances of an American heterosexual contracting AIDS are astronomical. They believe that they are safe; they are wrong. Probability statements can establish parameters of time and action within which a certain result is likely to occur. *If* you always flip a coin *exactly* the same way, *then* it is probable that *x* times it will come up heads and *y* times it will be tails. However, probability statements cannot tell you when the specific occasion of a head or tail may occur. You may get a run of 25 heads, followed by a run of 10 tails, or the two sides might alternate. The point is that no one can know whether the next flip will produce a head or a tail. Nor can anyone tell you whether the next sexual or drug encounter will be safe or not. Further, in real life there is much slippage in that word "exactly." These truths apply to the problem of describing how to avoid AIDS, just as they apply to flipping coins. The only honest response to the "Me worry?" reaction is to point out that people are dying within the odds. If it is sexual transmission, the very first encounter may be infectious, or it may be the 5000th, or never. There is no way to predict the safety of the individual event. If we could extrapolate from general odds to the specific occasion, no one would lose at Las Vegas.

Furthermore, probability statements are accurate only within strictly defined limits. Statisticians who project from existing data to future probabilities can only do so after assuring that their base data are accurate and timely, and only after prescribing certain constants or assumptions. The figure often seen in the press that 1.5 million Americans are infected with the virus is very suspect.[5] This estimate was projected from two sources: (1) an extrapolation from 1986 existing case data of about 30,000 cases and (2) a "guesstimate" based on Kinsey's 1940s estimate that about 10% of the American male population was dominantly or exclusively homosexual. If this remained the case in the 1980s, then it could be projected that about 10% of them would contract AIDS. The final figure of 1.5 million is, in other words, an estimate based on the current reported cases, plus an estimate based on 1940 data, and a certain assumed course of infection. It is no exaggeration to call it a "guesstimate."[6] In 1989 the California Medical Association estimated that there may be as many as 2.1 million seropositives in that state alone.[7]

A 1989 article in *Science* argued that the Centers for Disease Control estimates of seroprevalence levels among whites relative to ethnic minorities, and Midwesterners relative to Easterners, was much too low. The CDC answered that the methodology of the authors was flawed. The *Science* authors then countered with the projections of the Government Accounting Office, which suggested that they had, in fact, been gentle in their criticism of the CDC studies.[8] The CDC's estimates of the number of infected within the population has ranged from 650,000 to 1,500,000, while global estimates of the World Health Organization and other groups run from 10 to 15 million. The estimates will vary with the particular studies used, data comparisons, and the political climate. In the Reagan and Bush administrations there has been a tendency to downplay the epidemic, especially the extent of its intrusion into the middle-class heterosexual community.[9] If several possible figures are possible, announce the most optimistic one. Obviously, this eases the pressure on government to do something.

Part of the problem in getting a firm figure stems from the definition of AIDS. When you read that "$x\%$ of HIV+ will progress to AIDS within five years of primary infection," it is important to keep in mind that the statement does not say that you will get "sick" in five years, but that you will have developed the collection or syndrome of symptoms that the Centers for Disease Control have defined as constituting certifiable AIDS. This definition is very complex,[10] and just its revision in August 1987 produced a 20% increase in reported cases, both here and abroad.[11] It is quite possible to get sick and die of infections stemming from an HIV infection without, by definition, dying of AIDS. Epidemiologists estimate that there are more than *five times* as many individuals whose health is seriously impaired by HIV infection as there are those who have certifiable AIDS. Such individuals make up the large group of ARCs (people with aids-related conditions), who are sick and sometimes dying of "almost AIDS."[12] It is very likely that the official statistics on the epidemic, although grim, are not half grim enough.

Furthermore, many of the critical definitions that provide the foundation for projections and recommendations are themselves skewed and suspect. For example, our official reporting system for the spread of AIDS is based on questionable delineations of the groups involved. The IV drug user category is reasonably clear, but though it may seem extraordinary, it is nonetheless a fact that we do not have an acceptable definition of "straight" or "gay." There is good reason. Forty years ago Kinsey stated flatly that the population did not fall into these simple-minded categories:

> Males do not represent two discrete populations, heterosexual and homosexual. The world is not to be divided into sheep and goats. . . . It is a fundamental of taxonomy that nature rarely deals with discrete categories. Only the human mind invents categories and tries to force facts into separate pigeonholes. The living world is a continuum in each and every one of its aspects. The sooner we learn this concerning human sexual

behavior the sooner we shall reach a sound understanding of the realities of sex.[13]

Regardless of Kinsey's warning, the CDC uses such pigeonhole categories to report all data on the epidemic. Its *Morbidity and Mortality Weekly Reports* uses such categories as "homosexual," "bisexual," and "heterosexual" to organize and present figures on reported AIDS cases to the nation. All other discussion in the newspapers, on TV, and in the lecture hall relies upon these categories.

But who is "gay" and who is "straight"? The CDC classifies as heterosexuals only men who state that they have had no same-sex sexual encounters. A person is classified as homosexual or bisexual if he admits to any same-sex sexual activity. In all cases the reliability of the data depends upon candor, selective memory, and, above all, culturally determined perceptions of gender.[14] According to Kinsey 30% of the sexually active male population has had at least "incidental" homosexual experiences. The result, then, is that the CDC's heterosexual category applies to about 70% of the male, sexually active age group.[15] But it is a shifting or dynamic division, not a static one. As Kinsey put it,

> It is true that there are persons in the population whose histories are exclusively heterosexual. . . . And there are individuals . . . whose histories are exclusively homosexual. . . . But the record also shows that there is a considerable portion of the population whose members have combined . . . both homosexual and heterosexual experience and/or psychic response. There are some whose heterosexual experiences predominate, there are some who have had quite equal amounts of both types of experience.[16]

Can all the nuances that one finds in real life usefully be lumped into gross categories? Why, for example, should the "bisexual" be combined with the "homosexual" category: "homosexual and bisexual males"? Why not use the equally logical "heterosexual and bisexual males"? It is not at all clear whether the bisexual male is a homosexual who occasionally has sex with females, or a heterosexual who occasionally has sex with males.

It is all categorical nonsense. Being Haitian, "straight," or "gay," cannot be risky as such. HIV is spread by specific behaviors found to a greater or lesser extent in all groups; why not report in terms of known risky behaviors by whomever performed, such as anal sex?[17] The answer is that the categories have become partly political rather than purely epidemiological. In the early days of the epidemic the official risk classification system reflected the perception of the epidemic as the "gay plague." However, various projections of the American epidemic into the twenty-first century agree that it will become a predominantly heterosexual infection, just as it is already in

Africa and the Caribbean.[18] Then the heterosexual category will contain the chilling numbers; will it then become a "straight plague"? It is long past time to clean up the classification system so that sexually active people are given neither a false sense of security nor an equally false sense of despair, but are given full warning and guidance on what behavior to avoid.

HIV infection is clearly capable of being transmitted in several ways, but the virus itself is indifferent to the life-style preferences of the host. Reporting data in terms of the CDC classification encourages and perpetuates a misidentification of the essential problem. It focuses attention on more or less defined groups like gays or hemophiliacs. However, what is really important to us, as it is to the virus, is human behaviors, for some are much more apt to spread HIV than others. In discussing IV drug use and/or safer sex, it *is* important to know the kinds of behaviors to avoid; more often than not it is impossible to know what individuals to avoid.

Avoidance assumes that you have the necessary information to classify that person, and that the classification embodies a valid relationship. Ordinarily you do not. First, most of America's carriers are unaware of their condition. Second, a number of studies indicate that those who are aware are not eager to reveal their status. Lies not infrequently accompany the search for sex.[19] And finally, no one displays any outward sign of seropositivity until late in the course of the infection. If you have more money than good sense you can join a club that supplies a "Certified AIDS Free" membership card for use on dates. However, good sense requires that we discuss risk behaviors, not presumptively risky people.[20]

In other words, statistics and definitions have limitations, even when they come from authoritative sources like university research centers or the CDC. Many of the arguments in health and public policy stem from professional differences with regard to definitions and statistical methods. The sex researchers Masters, Johnson, and Kolodny challenge many of the figures, projections, and conclusions of the AIDS "establishment" in their book, *Crisis: Heterosexual Behavior in the Age of AIDS*. They argue that the official estimate of the infection's prevalence in the population is underestimated by about one-half, and that many public health conclusions (for example, that kissing is safe) are based on inadequate data.[21]

In addition, there are caveats that stem from the very nature of science itself and the business of data collection. The nonscientist must try to remember that the word *NEVER* does not exist in the vocabulary of laboratory science. The sun *might not* rise tomorrow, and you *might* get AIDS from the bananas packed for you by an infected grocery clerk, but these things have not, in fact, ever been recorded. I remember the head of the San Antonio AIDS Foundation losing his temper at a strategy meeting with physicians on just this point. The Foundation counselors were trying to determine what they should and should not say to people who called on the AIDS hotline for practical advice on how to avoid HIV infection. The scientists in attendance were hemming and hawing in their usual professional way when the Foundation president blew up and shouted, "How many centuries did it take for you guys to admit that people couldn't get syphilis from a toilet seat?" Silence reigned until someone sheepishly answered, "Oh, just one." Be that as it may, both the training and the philosophy underlying modern science absolutely rule out the "absolutely never."

Finally, there is a big difference between "hard" and "soft" data, and this difference frequently becomes critical in sensible discussions about AIDS-related behavior. Hard data are obtained when an observation embodies and reflects the use of commonly accepted and invariant standards—for example, when I state that this brick weighs 10 pounds. Others can check it out, weigh it themselves, and validate my data against a commonly accepted standard. This is "hard" data. There is precious little of it in the world of AIDS. What we generally have is indirect evidence, "soft" data, that is, data that may embody a person's judgment, cultural definitions, memory, or candor, or data that just seem to support the probability of a hypothesis. For example, one of the arguments for locating the geographic origin of HIV in central Africa is the very high rates of AIDS measured there. It seems a reasonable proposition that HIV must have been spreading a long time to establish such high rates of infection, and it had the time because it started there. Another example of "soft" data is found in statements made by interviewees in polls. Let us say that you want to know how many HIV+ males in Mexico City have seroconverted as a result of male-to-male sex. You conduct a poll, ask whether the interviewee is homosexual, and discover that 50% of the HIV+ will honestly answer no. You conclude that there must be a high rate of heterosexual seroconversion. But the conclusion may be wrong, because Latin males who are the active or insertive partners in male intercourse or oral sex do not consider themselves and are not considered by their culture to be homosexuals.[22] Epidemiologists, statisticians, and others go to great lengths to establish the reliability of their data, but inevitably their data gain authority through weight of numbers rather than conforming to a strict logical or standardized format, as in the case of hard data. Soft data are generally less precise and subject to more interpretation than is the case with hard data. How important this can be will be seen in the discussion below on the risks of oral sex.

Practicing physicians have their own set of professional limitations. A sense of limits flows from the fact that all competent physicians are painfully aware of how imprecise an art medicine really is, and equally aware of how much many patients emotionally need the assurance of a certain diagnosis. Thus, with one eye on medicine's limitations and the other on a possible malpractice suit, the physician prefers to say as little as possible and to state that little in very conditional terms.

Everyone wants clear, absolute, unambiguous statements from those perceived to have expertise. As far as HIV infection is concerned, no one is going to get them from honest sources. Like it or not, all that knowledgeable experts can endorse is behavior that will, with a little luck and in the greatest number of cases, enhance the chances of *avoiding AIDS*. Only idiots, charlatans, or con men will dispense prescriptions for something that does not exist—there is no absolute safety this side of Heaven.

AIDS AND IV DRUG USE

Obviously the most direct road to infection is direct injection of the virus into the bloodstream, the natural home of HIV. Acupuncture needles, blood transfusion needles, hypodermic syringes, and needles used to inject everything from antibiotics to heroin can accomplish this.[23] All that is required is that the needle be contaminated with the invisible virus. In the United States the likelihood of infection through a contaminated transfusion or the use of unsterile needles in a legitimate health care operation is too low (1:150,000–200,000) to be of concern from an epidemic standpoint. Accidents can and will happen that gravely concern the individual to whom they happen, but there will be too few to form the foundation of an epidemic endangering the nation.

Such is not the case with transmission of HIV through intravenous drug injection. The practices of 1.5 million IV drug users in the United States do pose a major hazard both to themselves and to the general community. The IV drug user subgroup has become a living storage reservoir for the virus, a source from which it is being transmitted to the greater community. IV drug users now account for about 30% of the total cases, and they are the major source of heterosexual and perinatal transmission.[24] The bridges are prostitution and the sale of blood to commercial plasma collection centers (*not* blood banks) by the addict.[25] There can be no battle to keep HIV out of the IV drug community; it is already well established, the virus having been introduced into the New York area drug community in the 1970s. Further, sometime in late 1987 data began to indicate that the rate of HIV infection in the groups practicing intravenous drug injection was increasing relative to those practicing anal intercourse. To put it another way, many of those practicing anal intercourse were getting the message about AIDS avoidance, but the IV drug user was not. The Surgeon General began warning that the control of AIDS in the future would be tied to the containment of IV drug use, and his warning was later echoed by Admiral Watkins, chairman of the Presidential AIDS Commission.[26] Unfortunately, these warnings have not yet registered at the White House. The National Commission on AIDS (the congressionally established successor to the Presidential AIDS Commission), in its December 1989 report, urged the President to take notice of this dangerous connection and revise the allocation of resources in his "war on drugs" to account for the AIDS/IV connection.[27]

Illustrative seroprevalencies within various IV drug subgroups are: San Franciscans enrolled in a community drug treatment program, 55%;[28] Chicago: west side, 30%, south side, 15.6%, and north side, 19.1%;[29] Manhattan clients of detox and methadone programs, 60%;[30] Atlanta clients of an STD center, 10%;[31] clients of a Puerto Rican drug treatment center, 45–59%;[32] and a small sample of Manhattan prostitutes, 50%.[33] The overall number of infected IV drug users in the United States is estimated to be 235,000 people, or 16% of the total. Most epidemiologists expect these figures, which are already on a par with those found in urban central Africa, to go up unless some way can be found to change patterns of drug use. Clearly, AIDS containment within the IV drug community is necessarily part of the larger "war on drugs" being waged by the Federal government.

After Teddy Roosevelt left the White House he went on an African safari and wrote a book on his prowess as a great white hunter. Illustrations showed Teddy standing on the carcass of an elephant, a dead rhinoceros, and other luckless animals that got in the way of his gunsights. With his usual flair and showmanship, he managed to convey the idea that the "Dark Continent" was forever illuminated by his brief sojourn there. But except for a few less animals, he left it as he found it. Somehow the Reagan-Bush "war on drugs" reminds me of Teddy's conquest of Africa. Newspapers showed Reagan's Attorney General Meese proudly standing in front of a pile of confiscated heroin. Nancy Reagan composed the administration's battle cry, "Just say no!," sweetly oblivious to the fact that the very nature of addiction is that you cannot just say no. President Bush, in an inspiring address on August 7, 1989, mobilized the Boy Scouts of America for the "war on drugs"; lots of showmanship but nothing really changes. The domestic and international drug industry continues to grow, increases its profits, and spawns ever more violence and destruction.

The interconnected wars to contain both the virus and IV drug use have many elements in common.[34] Winning them will be very expensive, although not as expensive in the long run as not winning them. Neither will be won without radical departures from currently acceptable approaches, nor will they be won without principled and courageous presidential leadership—the kind we associate with Abraham Lincoln. There is no likelihood, for example, that we will make a dent in the unbelievably lucrative drug traffic until the profit is taken from it. Americans should understand the power of the profit motive. That cannot be done by episodic, media-event drug raids or pious admonitions to middle-school students.

The national government could become the only legal supplier to those already addicted, combine free or low-cost supply with treatment programs for both addiction and AIDS if need be, and gradually (over the course of several generations) wean the commonwealth from its dangerous dependencies. Or on a less sweeping level, it could encourage shooting-gallery "house doctors" to promote the use of sterile needles. The cooperation of the "house doctors" (who are the shooting gallery experts at helping addicts find a usable vein) would have more effect on stemming the spread of AIDS via contaminated needles than all the press releases of former Secretary Bennett, the Bush administration's Don Quixote for drugs. Or the President could help sell the public on the notion that needle exchange programs are not designed to encourage drugs, but to discourage the spread of AIDS. If the President needs a national model to follow, he need look no farther than the Netherlands, Vancouver, British Columbia, or some American state programs. All of these programs treat the distribution of clean needles and condoms as equally important aspects of the fight to contain AIDS.[35] But if all of this is considered too radical for a national politician, a good deal of progress could be made simply by Congressional funding of existing drug treatment programs at the level called for by the population of IV drug users. Our programs can currently accommodate about 10% of the addicted population.[36]

SAFETY AND SEX

The necessary starting point for any discussion of safe sex is that there isn't any. There never has been. Sex and love have always been high-risk enterprises, as perhaps befits their centrality to the human experience. It has always been one of the main functions of both church and state to exert some control lest our hot pursuit damage the very community that our drives serve to perpetuate. From the days of Helen, whose face launched a thousand ships for the Siege of Troy, to the somewhat more mundane current possibility of contracting one of about 24 sexually transmitted diseases,[37] sex and love have been a problem—but one, I hasten to add, the burdens of which we have gladly assumed. Omar Khayyam, the great twelfth century Persian poet, immortalized our fantasies in his *Rubaiyat*:

> Here with a Loaf of Bread beneath the bough,
> A Flask of Wine, A Book of Verse—and Thou
>   Beside me singing in the Wilderness—
> And Wilderness is Paradise enow.

The Persian word for garden (*pardis*) is the source of our word *paradise*, a place of fulfillment, beauty, peace, a place to share with your beloved.

Gaining access to, retaining, and leaving a loved partner—one's microcosmic paradise—have always had a fatal potential. Indeed, most literature, poetry, and drama (as well as current TV soaps) revolve around the heady game. But always we have felt that the ultimate moment of passion and possession made the risks worthwhile. Now AIDS has dramatically upped the ante, and we are desperately searching for safer forms of sex.

What are the forms of safer sex in the context of AIDS, and what do I mean by "safer sex"? Safer sex practices are those for which there is no scientifically documented instance of seroconversion from negative to positive or where the evidence indicates a very low risk. By "documented" I mean findings corroborated by accepted scientific procedures sufficiently controlled to warrant being published in such reputable journals such as the *New England Journal of Medicine* and *The Journal of the American Medical Association*. There are now well over 160,000 cases of clinically recorded AIDS in the United States alone. These case records as supplemented by an impressive body of epidemiological evidence enable public health authorities to make recommendations that they would have hesitated to offer only a few years ago.

KISSING AND PETTING

As far as AIDS is concerned, kissing is safe—light or deep, on the cheek, on the hand, on the stomach, or wherever the spirit moves you. There are no documented cases of seroconversion attributable to kissing.[38] It is interesting to compare the U.S. government's brochures on avoiding AIDS in 1987 and 1988. The earlier cautioned against deep or "French" kissing, while the latter—mailed to the entire nation—stated flatly, "You won't get AIDS from a kiss."[39] Kissing is safe for several reasons. First, the virus apparently cannot penetrate unbroken outer skin layers (inner cervical or rectal membranes are another matter). Second, enzymes occurring naturally in saliva present the virus with a hostile environment, and stomach acids are fatal. Third, the infectivity of the virus is partially dependent upon its concentration in the fluid involved, and only very low quantities have been isolated from the saliva of even very advanced cases of AIDS.[40] Of course, there are always those who for reasons of private profit or fear will create theoretically dangerous scenarios. *If* you have an open sore on your lip or tongue, and *if* you let someone who is HIV+ chew on it for awhile, *then* seroconversion might possibly result. True. Anything is possible in this world; it is even possible that such people will grow up. But that possibility is probably much less than the chance of infection due to kissing. Unlike smoking, the Surgeon General has certified that kissing is *not* hazardous to your health.

On the other hand, kissing presents us with an excellent example of the difficulties in making unqualified recommendations when HIV is involved. While you will not be infected by the virus from kissing, you might get tuberculosis. People with HIV-damaged immune systems are susceptible to two forms of TB, one of which is transmissible by oral contact, coughs, and sneezes. It is not clear whether the increasing incidence of TB is the result of the activation of earlier infections or is the result of wholly new ones. Whichever, it is now recommended that all HIV+ individuals undergo annual TB skin tests and, if positive for TB, determine whether he or she is currently infectious. Fortunately, there is effective treatment; unfortunately, persistent coughing must now be regarded as a warning to affectionate friends and/or partners.

Other sexual expressions are without risk—hugging, cuddling, suppers by candlelight, the entire gambit of more exotic erotic fetishes (foot, clothing, pictures, etc.), pornography, cross-dressing, drag, massage and/or mutual masturbation, dancing, and hot tubs. The extraordinarily rich and imaginative array of behavior this side of intercourse are all still available as means of pleasuring your partner and yourself, of saying, "I love you, but am not willing to die for you." Once we get over being frightened by AIDS, we may find that it compels us to search our imagination for ways, other than ultimate ways, to express affection. We may even rediscover some past ways. A smart manufacturer could reproduce the colonial bundle-bed and bring old-fashioned country bundling back into vogue.

ORAL SEX

We have taken care of the lighter play. What about oral sex, sex involving contact between the mouth, the genitalia, the breasts, and other erotic zones. The signals from the research community are mixed on oral sex. Until very recently there has been no evidence whatever that HIV is transmitted through oral sex regardless of by whom performed, how performed, and on whom performed. Indeed, these findings so surprised researchers reporting in the British medical journal, *The Lancet*, that they made a point of mentioning what they had *not* found:

> The absence of detectable risk for seroconversion due to receptive oral-genital intercourse is striking. That there were no seroconversions detected among 147 men engaging in receptive oral intercourse with at least 1 partner . . . accords with other data suggesting a low risk of infection from oral-genital (receptive semen) exposure.[41]

No researcher has totally discounted the possibility, but it is fair to say that all the early American and English studies heavily discounted the probability of seroconversion through oral sex.

The team of Masters, Johnson, and Kolodny dispute these findings as, indeed, they dispute many current understandings relating to the transmission of HIV. With regard to fellatio, they argue that "there is no known viral or bacterial sexually transmitted disease that is not spread—at least at times—by oral-genital contact." Their point has a certain commonsense persuasiveness.[42] But they do not present data to sustain their position.[43]

However, in October 1989 San Francisco's health director, Dr. David Werdegar, announced that his researchers were "absolutely sure" that they had recorded two cases of seroconversion through oral sex. The evidence consisted of interview testimony.[44] This was followed a year later, in October 1990, by an announcement by Dr. Warren Windelstein, professor of epidemiology at the University of California's School of Public Health, that results of a study of 82 men in the Bay Area indicated that 17% seroconverted as a result of participating receptively in oral sex. The men in question denied that they had been involved in any other risk behaviors, such as anal intercourse or IV drug use.[45] If such data are ultimately found to be persuasive by the scientific community, the early understandings will have to be altered.

At this point it is important to recall previous comments with regard to hard and soft data. The new findings suggesting that oral sex presents a higher risk than previously believed necessarily rest on the accuracy of statements made by interviewees as to the character of their sexual behavior. More specifically, it turns upon their denial of acting as the passive or receptive partner in anal intercourse.

My experience at the San Antonio AIDS Foundation and my understanding of Western intellectual history lead me to advise great caution in accepting such denials. At the San Antonio AIDS Foundation, counselors have often seen initial denials retracted as the clients gained confidence in the discretion and caring of the counselors. Why should a man fervently deny being the passive partner in intercourse? Because an unbroken intellectual tradition, stretching back to Aristotle, condemns it as contrary to the "nature" of man. This view asserts that the male was designed to be the dominant, active sex; passivity or receptiveness would be, therefore, a perversion of the proper order of nature. Early Christian thinkers such as St. Paul and St. Augustine embellished Aristotle with assertions of a "natural" male superiority justified by their reading of scripture. Adam was, after all, first, and was made in the image of God. Both of them denounced men who allowed themselves to be used "as a woman" because it "lowers" a man, the original creation of God, to the lesser status of a woman.

These ideas became part of early church law and the general Western moral code. They remain powerful today, and can easily control verbal, if not always physical, behavior. It is not at all uncommon to encounter gay men, to say nothing of men who consider themselves straight, who refuse to admit to having—although they do not refuse to participate in—receptive anal sex. They too are hostages of the Western cultural tradition. It is easy for the scientist to overlook the awful, compelling power of our taboos because they are not readily measurable. Given the strength of data correlating receptive anal intercourse with HIV infection, given the paucity of data correlating receptive fellatio with infection, and given the power of the operating taboos, I would view statements denying anal sex with skepticism. Any study that finds an enhanced risk for oral sex on the basis of such denials must be examined with the greatest care. Each year thousands die of AIDS without being able to acknowledge the cause of their death even to relatives and friends. Similarly, I would wager, thousands become HIV+ without being able to admit to the behavioral source for their infection.[46]

Is oral sex risky or not? What is the answer? The answer is that, in the context of AIDS, the jury is still out. However, it has long since rendered the verdict with respect to other sexually transmitted diseases. Syphilis, gonorrhea, herpes, hepatitis B, various enteric diseases, and others are all transmitted through this practice, and there is some evidence that the microbes involved in these diseases can be cofactors in the transmission and/or activation of HIV. The United States is experiencing epidemic levels of these STDs as well as AIDS.[47] The bottom line is that, to be on the safer side, barrier protection from condoms or dams is indicated.[48]

SEXUAL INTERCOURSE

Last, but hardly least, is sexual intercourse, vaginal or anal. Sexually speaking, these practices are the high road to HIV infection, especially for the receiving or (badly mislabeled) "passive" partner. Both forms of intercourse have strong potential for transmission of HIV; either infected seminal fluid is ejaculated into the partner's body, or the penis is put in contact with infected anal or vaginal tissues and fluids. In either situation, the virus can then make its way from its point of origin into the recipient's bloodstream, either through ruptures in the interior linings or by direct interaction with mucosal cells.[49] The only access more direct to the bloodstream would be direct injection or transfusion with contaminated blood. The two modes of sexual intercourse do involve different public perceptions, resulting policies, and levels of risk.

Anal. If there is any subject that has ranked high on the list of America's nondiscussable subjects it is heterosexual or homosexual anal intercourse. In schools, Latin and Greek texts referring to this ancient sexual practice were left untranslated, mistranslated, or kept under lock in rare book rooms.[50] The fact that anal intercourse is one of the world's oldest and most widespread methods of birth control is largely ignored in America. The general American public attitude toward it is revealed by opinion polls indicating that many believe you can get AIDS through anal intercourse even though neither partner is infected with the virus![51] Only very recently (and as a result of the examination of our behavior forced by AIDS) is explicit American evidence surfacing. A letter published in the July 24/31, 1987, issue of the *Journal of the American Medical Association* indicates that as many as 25% of American women engage in some anal intercourse, and about 10% do so regularly. The conclusion was that "the number of women at risk through anal sex appears to equal the entire homosexual population of this country and exceed the number of homosexual men practicing receptive anal intercourse."

An ongoing study by Dr. David R. Bolling, Director of the Women's Health Center of San Antonio, Texas, indicated that 728 of the 1000 patients of the Center had tried anal intercourse and 238 of those (33%) were frequent participants.[52] In many Latin countries the possibility of exposure through anal intercourse is even more striking. The power of the Catholic church is such as to make condoms illegal or difficult to obtain, even if people wished to use them. In addition, the feudal-based tradition of machismo dictates that a woman be virginal upon marriage.[53] Both the requirements, of premarital birth control and maintenance of a technical virginity, are met through anal intercourse. In addition to heterosexual anal intercourse there is, of course, homosexual intercourse. There is no accurate measure of how many homosexuals participate in anal intercourse, both as active and passive partners, but it is probably a sizable majority. In any case the number of sexually active people involved is large, and all are participating in risky sex.

Wherever practiced and for whatever reason, the fact is that of the myriad sexual modes, anal intercourse carries the highest risk of infection for the receptive partner, regardless of that partner's gender. In the British study on this subject the investigators stated that "receptive anal intercourse was the only sexual practice shown to be independently associated with an increased risk of seroconversion to HIV in this study, and could account for nearly all new infections."[54] Similarly, an American study concluded that "The data . . . confirm that receptive anal/genital contact is the major mode of transmission of HIV infection."[55] However, neither study was able to establish that the insertive partner was at significantly enhanced risk of seroconversion;[56] in other words, the risk of transmission through anal intercourse is very asymmetric, and the receptive female or male bears most of the risk.[57]

Vaginal. The dominant practice of the dominant majority carries the third highest risk of seroconversion; only direct transfusion and anal sex outrank it. What are the odds? The answer is that there is no clear answer. Most studies that have dealt with vaginal-intercourse transmission from one partner to another have used as their original or "index" HIV+ partner someone who was infected by surgical or blood product transfusion. The results indicate that the rate of transmission is extremely variable, from 10% to 61%. This variability is also reflected in the data relating to the relative risk of the male and female partners. Some studies suggest that the risk is approximately equal or symmetrical, others that the female is at significantly higher risk.[58] The variabilities can be explained partly by differing methodologies and parameters, and significantly different target groups from "non-drug-using partners of IV users" to "wives of patients in Zaire." There are just not enough data on hand to be clear about the relative risks. A very theoretical study that received public attention in April 1988 stated that the chances of seroconverting as a result of one heterosexual encounter with someone who had tested free of the virus and during which a condom was used was 1 in 5 billion.[59] Other results from the same study indicated that the odds of seroconverting on the first encounter are 1 in 500 after engaging in condomless sex with an HIV+ partner and 2 out of 3 on or about the 500th.

Such findings are theoretically defensible, but no more useful than the statement, "It is highly improbable that you will be hit by a car while walking on an ice floe in the Antarctic." The authors of one of the studies mentioned above asserted that it was far more important that people chose partners carefully than that they avoid anal intercourse, use condoms, or limit their number of partners. More specifically, they advised that heterosexuals should protect themselves by having sexual relations only with partners they know to be in "low risk" groups, even though they acknowledge that this is difficult to know. Advice that cannot really be implemented is of questionable value. An individual can refuse receptive anal intercourse, insist on using condoms, and limit sexual partners, but just how does a person determine that the attractive someone is neither directly nor indirectly (through past or other partners) involved in a high-risk category?[60] The authors have fallen into the trap of which Kinsey warned. The world is not divided into sheep and goats; on the contrary, sexually it is a world where frequently one cannot tell the sheep from the goats.

SAFER SEX AND PUBLIC POLICY

Properly considered, the risk statistics should give little comfort to anyone. *Sex has become a zero-sum game, that is, EACH TIME you play you are in a win/no-win, all-or-nothing situation.* It is totally unlike playing the odds elsewhere. If you lose betting on the races or buying a Lotto ticket you can, with luck, recoup another day; *if you lose playing the AIDS odds, the loss is irreversible and irremediable, and your luck has completely run out.*

This harsh fact of life has many important implications for personal behavior as well as for government policy. For every individual it should rule out being the receptive partner in anal intercourse; all studies pinpoint this as the most dangerous sexual behavior. Regardless of gender, a personal policy of just saying no can, in fact, save your life.

On the public level we must learn to discuss the "unmentionables." One of the most extraordinary revelations brought about by AIDS is the depth of ignorance about the possibilities, functions, and dangers of sex. When I was a boy, a well-meaning adult sat me down and gravely informed me that my sanity would be endangered if I masturbated. He was wrong, but that was sex education in the early 1940s. The recently published *Kinsey Institute New Report on Sex* leaves the impression that the level of general understanding has not changed much since.[61] Alan Wabrek, president of the World Association for Sexology, lamented, "There is probably no other field of knowledge where, as a society, we even suggest that keeping people ignorant is the best policy."[62]

In San Antonio the Metropolitan Health District has made little headway in persuading the local school districts to implement meaningful AIDS avoidance education programs.[63] Except in the states most heavily affected by AIDS, colleges are not noticeably more enlightened. Some are now adding sexually transmitted diseases courses in recognition of the abysmal ignorance of the average first-year student. This is not to say that an 18-year-old does not know how to have sex; he or she most certainly does! Not a great deal of "education" is needed here. It means only that the entering student is blissfully ignorant of the implications and dangers that lurk in sex. Nonetheless, progress is slow; it is an uphill battle to get open and honest courses in the first- or second-year college curriculum. School superintendents and college presidents alike dread sparking religious controversies and are wary of the public relations impact on parents who, being parents (I do not exempt myself), prefer to think of their children as serious students rather than horny adults. The danger of these attitudes lies in the patent fact that the only thing more deadly than the virus itself is ignorance about it.

For its part, Congress continues to refuse funding for the national studies we need to get accurate information on American sexual behavior, and will only support the blandest of anti-AIDS public education campaigns. The distaste and denial associated with anal intercourse and its incorrectly exclusive association with homosexual behavior are so strong that it is difficult to have any dialogue. Public education campaigns that honestly and directly confront the real dangers are apt to be denounced by politicians and church leaders as pandering to "queers" and "sin," with predictably devastating results for funding. Even at the primary advising and care level, our taboos get in the way; it is often difficult to get AIDS counselors to raise the matter with clients, and the clients frequently do not want to hear.[64] Nonetheless, pious and ambiguous generalities are not strong enough to contain an epidemic.

In addition to avoiding anal intercourse, the number of sexual partners must be decreased, preferably to one. A point made strongly by most studies is that the risk of seroconversion is positively related to the number of different sexual partners. The subgroups within the San Francisco Men's Health Study displayed a range of seropositivity from 17.6% to 70.8%, depending upon the raw number of partners.[65] The results of the General Social Survey indicated that there were about 800,000 men in the United States, ages 18–44, who admitted to 10 or more partners in the preceding 12 months.[66] As in the case of receptive anal sex, the figures clearly point to sensible personal policy.

However, the public policy implications stemming from multiple-partners data are more complex and difficult. Should government promote the formation of loyal, monogamous relations and discourage incidental, transitory relationships? If so, how? Should it, for example, make possible homosexual marriage so as to introduce some legally backed stability into those relations? Homosexuals are frequently criticized for being "unstable" and promiscuous, but currently no state provides legal recognition for a stable homosexual union. Should government make divorce more difficult, or exert tighter controls on sexually explicit, fast-track advertising and programming? Currently our media glorifies a life style that is anything but an exemplar of stability, monogamy, and loyalty.

Any discussion of the multiple-partner problem must inevitably acknowledge the fact that America supports an enormous, varied, and thriving sex industry, from old-fashioned whorehouses, porno theatres, and sex shops, to so-called massage parlors, photo salons, dating clubs, baths, and singles bars, all of which promote transient contact and multiple exposures. Americans like sex; they just do not like to think about it. Different areas of the industry relate to the problem of containing AIDS in different ways. For example, if unbiased studies indicate that pornography is frequently used as a substitute for physical sex, and does not lead to interpersonal violence, then it would make sense for the national, state, and local governments to stop harassing the industry. On the other hand, a good argument can be made for closing or seriously regulating sex shops (as Nevada regulates prostitution), which provide the location and facilities for anonymous, fleeting homo- or heterosexual sex. The impact on the sustainability of the epidemic that results from the activities of a super-active subgroup who regularly patronize these businesses is substantial. James R. Thompson, professor of statistics at Rice University, calculated that:

if only 10 percent, say, of the gay community frequented bathhouses, *even if the less active members of the gay community decreased their contact rate in order that the same total number of contacts in the gay community was maintained,* it could have the same practical effect as would have been obtained if the entire gay community doubled their contact rate.[67]

Thompson argues that had the bathhouses been closed early in the epidemic, HIV's spread might have been significantly curtailed. Fear has now partially accomplished what public health authorities were reluctant to do years ago. However, this fear does not seem to have reached other parts of the country, or the heterosexual end of the business, even though its role in sustaining other STDs like herpes and gonorrhea is well documented.

A final point of agreement among the studies examining transmission is that the "proper use" of barrier latex condoms lessens risk.[68] But by how much? As with other information on sex, the data are scanty and ambiguous. The large statistical study referred to earlier assumed a 10% failure rate for condoms, a figure that manufacturers insist is too high. The Federal Drug Administration's inspection tolerance level is 4 defective (leaky) condoms per 1000, a standard that resulted in the rejection of many manufactured lots in 1987–1988. Condoms have been twisted, stretched, filled with water, blownup like balloons, and pumped in machines all in an effort to establish their reliability. They were even the subject of a major rating and testing article by *Consumer Reports* in March 1989.[69] All the data are necessarily inconclusive since none of the studies really field-test the device. What happens in the course of anal and vaginal intercourse is what is really important, not what happens in laboratory simulations of what happens in bed. Still, lab simulations, anecdotal review by users, and common sense are the best we are likely to get in this area. No one can argue that condoms provide complete protection; they do fail for various reasons and people have seroconverted in spite of consistent use.[70] On the other hand, rates of all sexually transmitted infections, including HIV, have dramatically decreased since 1982 within the San Francisco white, heterosexual population, and this decrease is attributed by researchers to sharply increased use of condoms.[71]

Data on adequacy aside, condoms are the only significant protection against the transmission of HIV during sex presently available. On the personal level common sense tells you that if seminal fluid is not deposited, it cannot infect.[72] On the public level, it seems reasonable to expect that a Congress that can rationalize the subsidy of tobacco farming could find the political courage to subsidize the distribution of life-saving condoms and encourage their use.

Avoiding AIDS

So, how does one avoid being infected with the Human Immunodeficiency Virus? From the viewpoint of both drugs and sex, the basic answer is, don't let it into your body.

If you shoot up the virus, you have committed suicide. Group use of syringes and needles is double dumb. Drugs are dumb to begin with; add HIV and unsterile works, and it totals double dumb. If hypodermic syringes are shared, then at least thoroughly cleanse and sterilize the works with a 1:10 solution of household bleach.

What is "safe" sex? The answer is that it is a wonderful, romantic myth. What is "safer" sex? Safer sex is first and foremost an attitude. It is the belief that you can give and receive love without endangering yourself or your partner, that there are emotionally satisfying exchanges short of sexual intercourse. The attitude that people have to "go all the way," to prove their masculinity, femininity, or commitment always was juvenile and risky, but it is now potentially fatal. Unless there is a change of our basic attitudes relating to sexual relations, the educational campaigns urging safer behavior are not apt to have much sustained effect.

As a behavioral matter, the answer to what is safer sex involves a combination of proscriptions and recommendations, and *they are the same regardless of gender or sexual disposition—straight, gay, bisexual, or whatever.*

But first I must make one exception. I do not believe that the concept of safer sex can apply to sexual relations between individuals, one of whom is known to be HIV+ and the other not, unless sexual intercourse and receptive oral sex are absolutely excluded. Omitting these sexual responses, there still remains a rich assortment of oral, visual, and tactile stimuli, including massage and masturbation. So the exclusion does not mean that one cannot have a loving, sexual relationship with an HIV+ partner; it means only that there ought not be a relationship involving penetration. There is nothing to be gained and much to be lost by ignoring the fact that penetrative sex with someone known to be HIV+ is a form of Russian roulette. The use of condoms does not change this perspective. First, in neither vaginal nor anal intercourse does the receptive partner have a reliable way of ensuring that a condom, or an effective condom is, in fact, being used. Checking in mid-course is not too likely. Second, even consistent use of condoms does no more than delay the inevitable; condoms do fail. Too many things can happen, and do.

The reality, however, is that in most cases, a person entering into intimate relations with another will ordinarily not have reliable information about the partner's HIV status. The partner may be genuinely HIV negative, may not

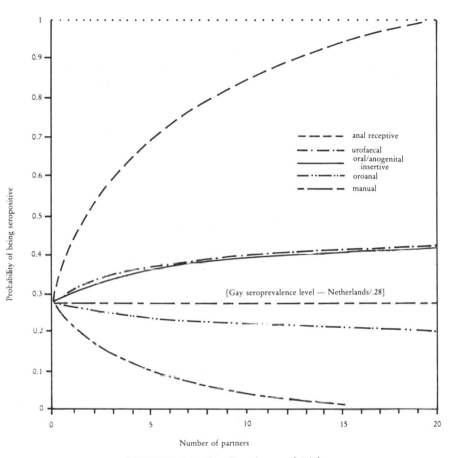

FIGURE 5.1   Sex Practices and Risk

Source: G. J. Van Greinfven, R. A. P. Tielman, and J. Goldsmit, "Prevalence of LAV/HTLV III Antibodies in Relation to Lifestyle Characteristics in Homosexual Men in the Netherlands" (paper presented at the International Conference on AIDS, Paris, June 1986), as reproduced in Tony Coxon, "The Numbers Game—Gay Lifestyles, Epidemiology of AIDS and Social Science," in Peter Aggleton and Hilary Thomas (eds.), *Social Aspects of AIDS* (London: Falmer Press, 1988).

know one way or the other, may be misinformed (as when he or she has tested negative, but falsely), or may lie. Under these circumstances the only reasonable course is to assume that the partner is a potential carrier and protect yourself either by abstention from the most intimate forms of sexual relations or by using such protection as has been demonstrated to offer good protection.

No form of sexual expression other than unprotected, condomless intercourse has been shown to present a major risk for the transmission of HIV.

Barrier protection with condoms or dams, especially if lubricated with products containing 65 mg nonoxynol-9, a spermicide toxic to HIV, reduce risk to acceptable levels.[73] By "acceptable level" I mean levels of risk lower than we assume in our daily lives without thinking much about it—the risk of a fatal auto accident, of sporting and gun accidents, and active and/or passive smoking, for example. Anal intercourse is extremely dangerous for the "passive" partner even with a condom, since condom failure is more likely in this mode.[74] Until a preventive vaccine is developed, receptive anal intercourse should be unequivocably excluded from everyone's portfolio of sexual expression. Vaginal intercourse is safer in that it is a less efficient mode of viral transmission and is less likely to produce condom failure. The risks involved in both forms become unacceptable if one partner has a sexually transmitted disease of any kind, but especially one that produces genital sores or lesions. If you see a sore or a rash, go no further. What evidence we do have indicates that oral sex is not an efficient means of transmitting HIV, but remember, it works just fine for everything else. So condom use is indicated here also. Finally, multiple partners and/or using any substance, like alcohol or drugs, to the point where your sense of self-preservation is dulled, enhances all risk, perhaps fatally.

The U.S. Public Health Service estimates that by the end of 1992 the Human Immunodeficiency Virus will have infected millions of Americans. The AIDS syndrone that terminates this infection will have killed 263,000 of us. It has also killed a game that millions once enjoyed, a game called "Casual Sex."

Notes

1. Except for the anchor categories, the ranking is approximate and suggestive only. Clearly, the transfusion of contaminated blood (no. 1) presents an almost 1:1 (95%) chance of infection. The chance of infection from blood bank supplies would depend upon the seroprevalence within the population of donors. In Zambia the chance would be high, in the United States low. For no. 11: The American Association of Blood Banks stated in 1989 that the chance of being infected by screened blood in the United States was between 1:100,000 and 1:200,000. Estimates as to the possibility of infection through unprotected anal intercourse (for the recipient partner) and medical accident like a needle stick from an HIV+ patient are both about 1:200.
2. Some of the variations, however, would not easily occur to someone not reading the literature. For example, a major concern has been the transmission of AIDS through the use of sperm, frozen or otherwise, dispensed from sperm banks. In October 1989 New York passed stringent new regulations requiring that sperm banks test donors twice in a six-month interval before their sperm was used in artificial insemination.

3. Robyn R. M. Gershon, David Vlahov, and Kenrad E. Nelson, "The Risk of Transmission of HIV-1 Through Non-Percutaneous, Non-Sexual Modes: A Review," from the Department of Environmental Health Sciences, and the Department of Epidemiology, The Johns Hopkins University School of Hygiene and Public Health, distributed by the Gay Men's Health Crisis, *AIDS Clinical Update*, October 1, 1990.

4. Uncircumcised men may be 5 to 8 times more likely to seroconvert from heterosexual intercourse than circumcised men; genital ulcers increase one's chances of seroconversion 4 to 5 times. See "Circumcision May Protect Against AIDS Virus," *Science*, August 4, 1989, p. 470.

5. For a good summary of the problems in arriving at accurate projections see "Projecting the Incidence of AIDS," *JAMA*, March 16, 1990, pp. 1538 *et seq*. On the original estimate of the Coolfont Planning Conference see M. I. Macdonald, "Coolfont Report: A PHS Plan for Prevention and Control of AIDS and the AIDS Virus," *Public Health Reports* 101 (1986): 341–48; and D. J. Bergman *et al.*, "Future Trends," same issue.

6. For a brief but very good discussion of the data reliability and projection problems see Peter Aggleton and Hilary Thomas, *Social Aspect of AIDS* (London: Falmer Press, 1988). Chapter 7, "The Numbers Game," deals specifically with the difficulties of getting reliable responses for statistical data on matters involving sex. The authors are generally, to put it mildly, very skeptical of the American data in general, and of the CDC reports in particular.

7. *Health InfoCom Network News*, October 16, 1989.

8. E. O. Laumann *et al.*, "Monitoring the AIDS Epidemic in the United States," *Science*, June 9, 1989. CDC's answers and the authors' counter-replies are in September 1, 1989 of *Science*. The General Accounting Office, in a backhanded swipe at the CDC estimates, suggested that perhaps the CDC needed a larger budget to expand its surveillance staff. See *National Journal*, July 1, 1989, p. 1715.

9. For a good review of the statistical problems and the understatements see William B. Johnston and Kevin R. Hopkins, *The Catastrophe Ahead* (New York: Praeger, 1990), chap. 3.

10. The definition used by the U.S. Social Security system and by the various state rehabilitation commissions in determining whether someone is eligible for AIDS disability financial assistance runs to six, double-columned, single-spaced pages of small print. More than one person living with AIDS has died before the bureaucrats could determine whether the individual was "sick" within the definition.

11. See various reports in *JAMA* 260, no. 15 (1988): 2213.

12. The ARC designation is now considered obsolete. Earlier it was thought that there might be a syndrome of conditions that would not necessarily progress to AIDS, and which could, therefore, be properly thought of as a separate set of ailments. It is now clear that this is not so.

13. Kinsey, Pomeroy, and Martin, *Sexual Behavior in the Human Male* (New York: Saunders, 1948), p. 19. And see Kinsey, et al., *Sexual Behavior in the Human Female* (New York: Saunders, 1953).

14. For example, if you tell a Latin American, Caribbean, Mediterranean, Middle Eastern, or Azerbaijani male that he is "gay" because he has a male lover, you may provoke a dangerously violent reaction in defense of his machismo or

honor. Those cultures limit the idea of homosexuality to the so-called passive partner. AIDS workers quickly discovered this in San Antonio, where a HIV+ Puerto Rican emigré may have both male and female sex partners and be considered absolutely straight—so long as he is the dominant or active partner.

15. Kinsey, Pomeroy, and Martin, *Sexual Behavior in the Human Male*, p. 25.
16. Ibid., p. 19.
17. The model for projecting AIDS cases developed by mathematician Yakov Fuxman takes this approach. His model reflects individual risk factors, rather than categorized groups. For that reason it projects farther into the future and more accurately. See Rebecca Voelker, *American Medical News*, December 22, 1989, p. 4.
18. For example, see the scenarios portrayed in Johnston and Hopkins, *The Catastrophe Ahead*, pp. 137–46.
19. Susan D. Cochran and Vickie Mays reported on their studies on this matter in the correspondence section of the *N. Engl. J. Med.*, March 15, 1990, p. 774. Their general conclusion was that a sizable percentage of college-age, sexually active students (more men than women) do not tell the truth about their sex lives to their partners.
20. Across the United States and the world there is a significant variation in population seroprevalence. The New York–Washington–Boston population corridor has the highest seroprevalence rate in the nation, with the South Bronx the highest within that area. On the other hand, North Dakota is, so far, relatively untouched by the epidemic. The entire picture, then, relates both to what you do and where you do it.
21. Masters, Johnson, and Kolodny, *Crisis: Heterosexual Behavior in the Age of AIDS* (New York: Grove Press, 1988), Chaps. 1 and 2.
22. See the story filed by Nancy Nusser from Mexico City, Cox News Service, "AIDS on Increase; Gays Ignore Risks," *San Antonio Express-News*, September 16, 1990, p. 2G.
23. An acupuncture case was reported from France. See *N. Engl. J. Med.*, January 26, 1989, p. 250.
24. See the study and its citations, Jordan B. Glaser and J. Strange, "Heterosexual Human Immunodeficiency Virus Transmission Among the Middle Class," *Archives of Internal Medicine* 149 (March 1989): 645–49.
25. "Drug Abusers with AIDS Virus Are Selling Plasma, Study Finds," *New York Times*, April 25, 1990, p. A10, reporting on a Johns Hopkins School of Hygiene and Public Health study that documented that 23% of 2921 IV drug users surveyed in the Baltimore area in 1988 and 1989 said that they had sold plasma or donated blood after they began IV drug use.
26. See *Wall Street Journal*, February 28, 1988, p. 24E.
27. The National Commission was so disturbed that it took the unusual step of issuing a preliminary report eight months earlier than mandated by the congressional act creating it.
28. Heterosexual i.v. drug users enrolled in a San Francisco drug treatment program. Richard E. Chaisson *et al.*, "Cocaine Use and HIV Infection in Intravenous Drug Users in San Francisco," *JAMA*, January 27, 1989, pp. 561–65.
29. See "Study of IV Drug Users and AIDS Finds Differing Infections Rate, Risk Behaviors," *JAMA*, December 2, 1988, p. 3105. "Links between Cocaine and Retroviral Infection" (editorial), *JAMA*, January 27, 1989, pp. 607–8.
30. Don C. Des Jarlais *et al.*, "HIV-1 Infection among Intravenous Drug Users in

Manhattan, New York City, from 1977 through 1987," *JAMA*, February 17, 1989, pp. 1008–12.

31. Robert A. Hahn *et al.*, "Prevalence of HIV Infection among Intravenous Drug Users in the United States," *JAMA*, May 12, 1989, pp. 2677–84.

32. Ibid., p. 2679.

33. Ibid.

34. See D. C. DesJarlais and S. R. Friedman, "AIDS and IV Drug Use," *Science*, August 11, 1989, p. 578. The authors point out that the drug problem is really not *one* problem; there is considerable variation to be found within the total group that uses intravenous injection. In Sweden, for example, 50% of the heroin users are HIV+, while only 5% of the amphetamine injectors are. Why? Similarly, the seroprevalence rate among IV users in New York City is 50%, in San Francisco 15%, and in Los Angeles 5%. Again, why the differences?

35. Michael Gray, "Fighting AIDS with Needle Exchanges," *American Medical News*, February 16, 1990, p. 33 *et seq*. On the Vancouver program see *New York Times*, April 17, 1990, p. A7.

36. See the testimony of Dr. Evridiki J. Hatziandreu, Congressional Office of Technological Assessment, *New York Times*, September 19, 1990, p. A12.

37. Alan R. Hinman, MD, Director of the Division of Sexually Transmitted Diseases, Centers for Disease Control, *Sexually Transmitted Diseases Treatment Guidelines, 1989* (Washington, DC: Public Health Service, MMWR series 38, no. S-8, October 1989).

38. Masters, Johnson, and Kolodny in *Crisis* argue that the data is inadequate on this point due to the fact that kissing as a form of sexual behavior is not behaviorally or statistically isolated from other forms occurring simultaneously, and therefore it is not possible to conclude that transmission of virus did not occur from kissing. The problem they raise bedevils the entire area of AIDS research and the recommendations coming from it. The inevitable ambiguities are exploited by those who advocate a use of mandatory testing, contact tracing, and quarantine in the AIDS epidemic. See, for example, the upscale, "yuppie" approach to promoting a homophobic, fundamentalist epidemic control agenda in *New Dimensions* 4, no. 3 (March 1990).

39. Compare Otis R. Bowen, M.D., Secretary of the Department of Health and Human Services, *What You Should Know About AIDS* (U.S. Public Health Service, Centers for Disease Control, 1987), with C. Everett Koop, M.D., Surgeon General of the United States, *Understanding AIDS* (Washington, D.C.: U.S. Government Printing Office, Public Health Service, Centers for Disease Control, 1988).

40. P. C. Fox, A. Wolff, C. K. Yeh *et al.*, "Saliva Inhibits HIV-1 Infectivity," *Journal of the American Dental Association* 116 (1988): 635–37; P. N. Fultz, "Components of Saliva Inactivate HIV," *The Lancet* 2 (1986): 1215.

41. Lawrence A. Kingsley, Richard Kaslow *et al.*, "Risk Factors for Seroconversion to Human Immunodeficiency Virus among Male Homosexuals," *The Lancet*, February 14, 1987, p. 348. The *Lancet* study confirmed an earlier one reported in the *Journal of The American Medical Association*: Warren Winkelstein, *et al.*, "Sexual Practices and Risk of Infection by the Human Immunodeficiency Virus: The San Francisco Men's Health Study," *JAMA*, January 16, 1987, p. 321. Also see D. Lyman *et al.*, "Minimal Risk of Transmission of AIDS-Associated Retrovirus Infection by Oral-Genital Contact," *JAMA*, 255 (1986): 1703. A. R. Lifson, "Do Alternate Modes for Transmission of Human Immunodeficiency

Virus Exist?" *JAMA* 259 (1988): 1353–56. The author, Alan Lifson, M.D., M.P.H., is an epidemiologist at the Federal Centers for Disease Control working at the San Francisco Department of Health.

42. One researcher contends that the data used by Masters *et al.* do not support their arguments. See E. H. Kaplan, "Crisis? A Brief Critique of Masters, Johnson and Kolodny," *Journal of Sex Research* 25, no. 3 (August 1988): 317–22. And see *AIDS Alert, The Monthly Update for Health Professionals* 3, no. 2 (April 1988), an issue in which the authors of some of the research studies cited by Masters deny that their work is being properly used by the authors.

43. Masters, Johnson, and Kolodny, *Crisis*. And see "Transmission of HIV Infection from a Woman to a Man by Oral Sex" (correspondence), *N. Engl. J. Med.*, January 26, 1989, p. 251. Two clinicians associated with the Lahey Clinic Medical Center of Burlington, MA, report what they believe to be the first documented case of seroconversion due to oral sex.

44. Associated Press dispatch, October 12, 1989, *Science/Medicine AIDS Newsgroup* (distributed electronically through the InterUniversity BITNET system).

45. See the Associated Press release of October 7, 1990, "AIDS by Oral Sex Higher than Expected," *San Antonio Express-News*, October 7, 1990, p. A1. There have been other clinical and anecdotal indications of some risk, but none of sufficient persuasiveness to dislodge the earlier consensus that oral sex presented a risk so low as to be negligible.

46. A British social scientist states flatly that "studies of the *reliability* of self-reports of sexual behavior show that, in general, the retrospective recall of information tends to be selective, ordinally distorted and unreliable" (my emphasis). See Tony Coxon, "The Numbers Game—Gay Lifestyles, Epidemiology of AIDS and Social Science," in Peter Aggleton and Hilary Thomas (eds.), *Social Aspects of AIDS* (London: Falmer Press, 1988), p. 129.

47. Rebecca Voelker, "STDs Near Epidemic Levels, Experts Agree," *American Medical News*, June 2, 1989, p. 3. According to the testimony, the United States has experienced a 67% increase in hepatitis B since 1978, and now has about 30 million cases of genital herpes. Both of these VDs are clearly implicated in the spread of HIV.

48. Apart from the risk of disease transmission, it might be noted that sodomy can be legally risky. In about one-half the states it is illegal. A Maryland trial judge in 1988 imposed a five-year prison sentence upon Steven Schochet for having oral sex with a woman to whom he was not married. The sentence was upheld by the state court of appeals, citing as authority the United States Supreme Court's decision in *Bowers v. Hardwick*, 487 U.S. 186 (1986), a case that upheld Georgia's sodomy laws as applied to homosexuals.

49. "The Transmission of AIDS: The Case of the Infected Cell" (commentary) *JAMA*, May 27, 1988, p. 3037.

50. Peter Fryer, *Private Case—Public Scandal* (London: Secker & Warburg, 1966).

51. June M. Reinisch, with Ruth Beasley, *The Kinsey Institute New Report on Sex: What You Must Know to be Sexually Literate* (New York: St. Martin's Press, 1990).

52. See the discussion, "Sex Experts and Medical Scientists Join Forces against a Common Foe: AIDS," *JAMA*, February 5, 1988, pp. 641–43.

53. This was rationalized in terms of the man's honor but, in fact, had more to do with maintaining the lines of descent that established, in a feudal society, claims

over property and power. The church elaborated rules of legitimacy to clarify lines of descent and thereby stabilize property relations and control from the king on down. The alternative was civil strife. Premarital pregnancy as well as adultery were intolerable because they both confused and endangered orderly succession to property and power. Prospective queens had to be virginal and were examined to make sure they were. Adultery with a queen was high treason. The king could sire illegitimate children without endangering the legitimate succession to the throne, but the queen could not, because only she could, as it were, palm off her child as the child of the king and legitimate heir to the throne. In illegitimacy lay the beginnings of civil war in a feudal monarchy.

54. Lawrence Kingsley *et al.*, "Risk Factors for Seroconversion," *The Lancet*, February 14, 1987, p. 347.

55. Warren Winkelstein *et al.*, "Sexual Practices and Risk of Infection," *JAMA*, January 16, 1987, p. 324. See also "The Transmission of AIDS," (commentary), *JAMA*, May 27, 1988, p. 3037.

56. The only study I have seen that attempts to establish rough quantitative relationships between active or "insertive" anal intercourse and probability of seroconversion is found in Aggleton and Thomas, *Social Aspects of AIDS*, pp. 136–37.

57. The data, especially from Africa, indicate that the insertive partner is at high risk of acquiring infection from an infected partner if the insertive partner has genital sores (as from herpes infection), which can act as a portal for the virus. Apparently, uncircumcised men are also at higher risk.

58. Thomas A. Peterman *et al.*, "Risk of Human Immunodeficiency Virus Transmission from Heterosexual Adults with Transfusion-Associated Infections," *JAMA*, January 1, 1988, pp. 55–58. "The Transmission of AIDS: The Case of the Infected Cell," p. 3037. Editorial, *JAMA*, October 7, 1988, p. 1943.

59. Norman Hearst and Stephen Bailey, "Heterosexual AIDS," *JAMA*, April 22, 1988.

60. On the point, "How do you know?", see the very interesting discussion in *JAMA*, October 7, 1988, pp. 1879–91.

61. Reinisch and Beasley, *The Kinsey Institute New Report on Sex*.

62. Quoted in *San Antonio Express-News*, October 16, 1990, p. 13A.

63. "Lack of AIDS Teaching Rapped," *San Antonio Express-News*, October 6, 1990, p. 8B.

64. This problem is not unique to America, by any means. See Rachel Sternberg, "Fighting Taboos, Fighting AIDS—Mexican Health Officials Focus on Prevention," *American Medical News*, February 3, 1989. The Muslim Middle East is another area where religious and cultural taboos get in the way of accurate reporting and counseling.

65. Winkelstein, "Sexual Practices and Risk of Infection," *JAMA*, vol. 257, no. 3, (1987) p. 321. But it is not a simple matter. Multiple exposures and multiple partners are different matters and are frequently difficult to disentangle. Nonetheless, the conclusion stated by one group contains a strong implied warning and recommendation, "As infectivity estimates are revised upward or as variable infectivity levels become significant, the risk associated with multiple sexual partners increases." D. P. Francis and J. Chin, "The Prevention of AIDS in the United States," *JAMA*, vol. 257 (1987), p. 1357, and *JAMA*, October 7, 1988, p. 1879.

66. "Leads from the Morbidity and Mortality Weekly Report, Centers for Disease Control," *JAMA*, October 14, 1988, p. 2020.

67. James R. Thompson, "Taking Sides, AIDS: Old Disease, New Society," *This Side of Rice*, April–May 1988, p. 12. This publication circulates mainly at Rice University. For more accessible statements on the AIDS epidemic by Professor Thompson see "AIDS: The Mismanagement of an Epidemic," *Computers and Mathematics with Applications*, vol. 18, (1989), pp. 965–72, and "A Simple Model of AIDS," in *Empirical Model Building* (New York: John Wiley, 1989).

68. It is important to specify "proper" in this context. First, the condom must be put on correctly to minimize the possibility of breakage, with no captured air bubbles except at the tip. Second, it must be of the latex variety and not be lubricated with petroleum-based products, which cause the latex to break down quickly. Water-based lubricants with nonoxynol-9 are preferred. Third, condoms must be used consistently to have any significant statistical safety advantage; just "once in a while" will not do.

69. "Can You Rely on Condoms?" *Consumer Reports*, March 1989, pp. 135–41.

70. See William B. Johnston and Kevin R. Hopkins, *The Catastrophe Ahead*, pp. 70–72 on condoms, and the references cited there.

71. Centers for Disease Control Reports, "Current Trends: Heterosexual Behaviors and Factors that Influence Condom Use among Patients Attending a Sexually Transmitted Disease Clinic—San Francisco," *Morbidity and Mortality Weekly Report*, October 4, 1990.

72. A point of clarification: Sperm itself is not the villain in spreading HIV; rather, it is spread as free virus particles or virus-carrying white blood cells found in semen. See "Do Sperm Spread the AIDS Virus?" *Science*, July 7, 1989, p. 30.

73. Eve K. Nichols, *Mobilizing against AIDS* (Washington, DC: NAS, rev. ed., 1989), p. 150.

74. G. J. Van Greinfven, R. A. P. Tielman, and J. Goldsmit have plotted curves comparing the probability of seroconversion as functions of type of sex and number of partners. Anal intercourse stands out dramatically as the most dangerous practice. See Aggleton and Thomas, *Social Aspects of AIDS*, pp. 136–137, which discusses and reproduces the curves presented in the original Van Greinfven report (Van Greinfven, "Prevalence of LAV/HTLV III Antibodies in Relation to Lifestyle Characteristics in Homosexual Men in the Netherlands," paper presented to the International Conference on AIDS, Paris, June 1986).

6

===

The Infected Body Politic

All natural disasters, be they earthquakes or epidemics, place the individual and the commonwealth under a multitude of strains. Some, like earthquakes or a firestorm of flu, are mercifully fast. After the event the nation pulls itself together, swings into action to clean up damage, bury the dead, and hopefully to install controls to ameliorate the cost in lives and treasure of the next episode—for there is always a next episode. Other peoples around the globe rally with assistance; all understand that "There, but for the grace of God. . . ." The recent earthquakes that devastated Mexico City, Soviet Armenia, and the San Francisco Bay Area come to mind.

However, AIDS is a catastrophe of a compellingly different kind. It did not strike like a snake; rather, it burrowed (and continues to burrow) insidiously like a giant mole under the walls of the republic, undermining lives and challenging the genuineness and solidity of our social, economic, and political commitments. It had already done enormous damage before the nation became aware of its existence. Between 1980 and 1983 a few coura-geous and prescient individuals like Dr. Max Gottlieb at UCLA, playwright Larry Kramer in New York, and journalist Randy Shilts in San Francisco warned of the danger, but their calls of alarm were lost in a wilderness of disbelief, denial, and inertia.

This was the time, the early 1980s, when AIDS and its costs might have been contained, but effectively raising the alarm entailed serious political risks in all the affected communities—the political, the religious, and the homosexual. Political and religious leaders took their cue from President Reagan's deafening silence, and most national, state, and local public and private institutions dithered through the critical years.

The lack of leadership can be attributed to many perfectly ordinary and understandable human reactions. There is a natural tendency to ignore bad news and hope that "it" will go away, or "it" will turn out to be nothing more than a recapitulation of the embarrassingly baseless swine flu scare of

President Ford's administration. Until his friend Rock Hudson died in 1985, President Reagan apparently thought of AIDS as something like a passing epidemic of measles.[1] And clearly, within the highest ranks of the establishment there was a general lack of sympathy for and sense of community with those who were the main victims in the early years.

However, in fairness it must be admitted that the establishment's policy of not-so-benign neglect was matched by the myopia of gay leadership. Effective action from within the nation's various gay communities, the communities most affected in these early years, was severely hampered by a Gordian knot of self-doubt and denial. Homosexuals are not immune to the perception of them encountered in the heterosexual mainstream. Indeed, most of the culture's homophobic attitudes are internalized in the homosexual; the victim is taught to believe in the essential rightness of his oppressor's position.[2] Perhaps, after all, the epidemic *was* a plague sent by God. I remember an 18-year-old client of the San Antonio AIDS Foundation saying to me one day, "I know that I have to bear this as well as I can. I got it because I was playing around, and God is punishing me." I wondered how one so young could believe that his life, barely under way, was so corrupt and sinful as to deserve such a fate; he hadn't even had the time to become a proper sinner. I was about to argue with him when it occurred to me that maybe it is better to die with some personally plausible explanation than to die for no apparent reason at all. In addition, the gay leadership in such cities as San Francisco and New York feared that acknowledging that there was a connection between aspects of the male gay life style and viral spread would invite a majority backlash, wiping out their recent gains in establishing community identity and autonomy.[3]

For all these reasons and more, the virus went relatively unchallenged during its first years in America; it took a deep and firm hold. Too many of our political, religious, and economic leaders, both gay and straight, turned their backs on the afflicted and ignored the epidemic as long as they could. Now all of us will pay the bill for their failure of conscience and negligence. Here and abroad, the costs will now be beyond measure.

The American philosopher George Santayana once said, "Those who do not remember their past are condemned to repeat it." Now we must relearn a lesson our ancestors of the Civil War learned the hard way, that we all live in one house; what destroys some of us threatens all of us. We cannot isolate ourselves from the spread of the virus and the multitude of effects that follow in its wake; we cannot run to the country as people did in the days of the bubonic plague. We are an urban civilization and the viral carrier lives next door. As a united people we will contain this dreadful epidemic. If we continue to divide along class, life-style, ethnic, or religious lines, HIV will undermine the health of our republic as surely as it does the lives of its individual citizens.

THE CORROSION OF GRIEF

Generations ago an action for damages could be filed for the emotional injury that resulted from being left at the altar. It was the action for breach of promise to marry. Gilbert and Sullivan, in their own inimitable way, lampooned it in *Trial by Jury*. It is no longer recognized as an independent cause of action, not because the injury is unreal or insubstantial, but because we concede that the injury is not subject to the quantitative measure that modern judges and juries insist upon before awarding compensatory damages. Everyone who has lived a little can testify that emotional injury is very real and that grief is debilitating. But how much is the injury worth in cold cash, in hard dollars? It is all too subjective and ambiguous, too difficult to produce reasonable evidence; our legal system tends to break down when confronted with such intimate matters. It is somehow ironic that we can measure the weight of cosmic dust falling upon the earth or the dimensions of an infinitesimally small expression of nature like the human immunodeficiency virus, but cannot measure the value or weight of the universally experienced phenomenon of human grief. But measure or not, we owe it to those who have died, and will die, in this epidemic to acknowledge their suffering. Properly, we must pay them homage for being the source of knowledge that may save future generations of maturing, sexual adults from the horror of AIDS.

Even if we cannot measure our sorrow, we can express it. Indeed, to stay healthy, we must express it. AIDS is inspiring a whole new aesthetic of grief in plays, stories, visual art, and dance.[4] It has also inspired one of the most moving memorials created in our time, the AIDS Memorial Quilt. It is an enormous patchwork quilt composed of over 14,000 coffin-sized panels bearing the names of those who have died of AIDS, portions of which tour the nation. It is comparable only to the Vietnam War Memorial in Washington, DC. The War Memorial was erected by a nation grieving its dead and, perhaps even more, the death of its delusions of global invincibility. The Quilt is being sewn by grieving parents, spouses, lovers, and friends to express their grief. Some representative panels of the Quilt have now been added to the collection of the Smithsonian. Whether on display as a public monument or as an artifact of grief in the "nation's attic," the two are similar in that they are composed of names, and names, and more names; names of people killed in war, names of people killed in an epidemic, all of them together now in the equalitarian commonwealth of death. But there is also a melancholy difference between the two. The Vietnam Memorial, with its almost 60,000 names, is finished. The Quilt will not be completed in our time, for the epidemic marches on and the list gets longer. In a scant 20 years a complete quilt might well require 7 million panels in America alone![5]

It seems to me that the pain and suffering following in the wake of AIDS

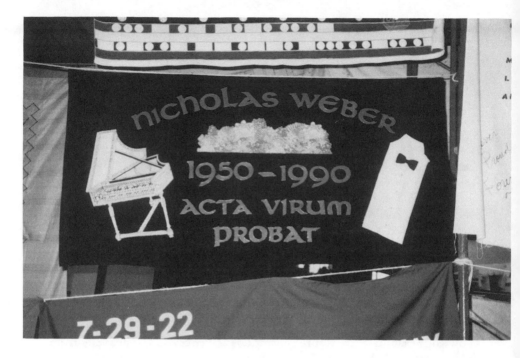

FIGURE 6.1   Panel from the AIDS Memorial Quilt: Nicholas Weber,
Harpsichordist and Composer, Panel 0155–6

have some qualities with which it is especially hard to cope, and which set it
apart from other disasters. First, AIDS strikes hardest at the young adult; it
cuts people down in the full vigor and bloom of their youth. Those who care
for AIDS patients testify that this is the most demoralizing aspect of their
work, with emotional burnout a constant hazard because of it.[6] There was
an elderly 70-year-old AIDS patient named Jake at the hospice where I
volunteer. He was a wonderful, if sometimes irascible old gentleman who
put up with little nonsense from the many younger clients of the Foundation. He could soundly whip all of them at any game of cards and would
occasionally condescend to teach the skills of bridge or poker. All of the
volunteers were concerned about Jake, but somehow it was not the same as
their concern about the younger clients. We did not want Jake to suffer, we
wanted him to be as comfortable as possible, but the greater measure of grief
was reserved for the 20-year-old to whom he was teaching poker. We knew
that Jake's students would never really have the opportunity to practice and
hone their new skill the way Jake had over a long lifetime. I think we all

instinctively understand that it is the younger age group that holds the future of the nation in its hands; there is an enormous difference between our emotional reaction to someone dying after almost three-quarters of a century of living and one who is just beginning.

A second difficulty lies in the fact that, for the foreseeable future, there is no closure to the epidemic nor to the grief that it will cause. In war a person is killed, we conduct rites, we bury, and eventually the pain subsides to manageable proportions. There is closure. Only for those unfortunate people whose loved ones are still Missing in Action is there a special kind of continuing grief, precisely because the books cannot be closed; there is no finish, no closure. The great epidemics of the past took their toll and burned themselves out; we portrayed these deadly events as an arrival of the Grim Reaper who, with the scythe of death, mowed broad swaths through fields of people. But as reapers do, he moved on. Now, with AIDS he proposes to stay a while—at least into the twenty-first century—as a major partner in our lives and loves.

Third, these problems are worsened by the fact that AIDS is a diabolically deceptive disease with a long season of dying. Those who are infected may present no outward sign of the affliction for many years. Then when they start to show their illness, they frequently look and feel fine one month only to look and feel sick the next. The up periods generate false hopes that are dashed to bits by the following down stage. The erratic character of the affliction, together with the long period of general decline, can find everyone, patient and survivor alike, silently praying for death, for closure at the end.

Finally, the plague mentality endemic to our religious and cultural traditions makes it difficult for survivors to confide in and get necessary support from the circle of relatives and friends who ordinarily would be there for them. There is widespread concealment and deception on both the personal and public levels. Frequently the shame of dying from AIDS affects patients so strongly that they delay notifying parents until the last minute, if at all. In my experience, the parents usually rally to the support of their afflicted children no matter what, but they often find themselves very much alone with the problem. They do not feel as though they can confide in their relatives and friends to gain the emotional support they need. The best known instance of attempted concealment was Rock Hudson's attempt to keep the information from his lover and the public. His action formed the basis of the successful damage suit against his estate. One of the striking evidences of the stigma's power can be seen in the obituary columns. In San Antonio there have been well over 300 deaths from AIDS, but there have been only two or three obituaries that indirectly indicated the cause.

None of us can live with active, corrosive, gnawing grief indefinitely. We need to put an end to it and get on with the business of living. Elizabeth Kübler-Ross' famous five stages of dying (denial, anger, bargaining, depression, and acceptance) apply not only to the patient, but also to the patient's surviving spouse, lovers, parents, and friends. I have frequently witnessed them going through the same process, especially the bargaining stage. But for survivors there must be one more stage; between depression and acceptance there must be closure, for without it there is no acceptance. Twenty-five hundred years ago the Greek dramatist Sophocles had his heroine, Antigone, challenge King Creon in order to bury her fallen warrior brother. Creon's decree, denying him a soldier's burial, condemned his spirit to wander hopelessly forever, a tormented shade upon the Earth. Antigone, in one of the great speeches of all drama, indicted Creon for violating the eternal laws of nature, laws which not even a king could change. Defying the king, she buried her brother to give peace to his soul and rest to her grief.[7]

But kings can be defied with more effect than disease. AIDS will give us no quick closure, no respite; it will test our capacity for compassion and grief. Many of us will try to deny, discount, and ignore it rather than confront and contain it. This is natural. This is understandable. It is also futile. In the end avoidance behavior will just prolong the agony, as well as enhance the guilt that all survivors feel who have failed to do what they could. The only way we can achieve closure, to close the books on grief, is to satisfy ourselves that we have cared for the afflicted with love and compassion, that we have done what we could do. Like Antigone, we must do our duty, do what is right, both for our own peace of mind and for the souls of our fallen kindred.

PROFIT AND LOSS

It sounds almost obscene to utter the phrase "profit and loss" in the context of such a human calamity, but if we are looking at the costs of AIDS, utter it we must. Montaigne, in one of his shortest essays, reminds us that "no profit is made save at a loss to someone else."[8] AIDS is a natural biological event just as an earthquake is a natural geological event. It is a devastating psychological event with both individual and group impact. It is a religious event with potential for both the stimulation of future good as well as the rekindling of past evil. It is also a politico/economic event of stupendous magnitude.

Anne Skitovsky, an expert in health economics, estimated that by 1991 the national economy will have to absorb a $55 billion annual loss in productivity attributable to illness and premature death due to AIDS.[9] The figure is higher than might otherwise be the case due to the fact that AIDS strikes most vigorously at those between 20 and 40, the age group that in gross terms is the most productive. However, the $55 billion figure is actually a very low estimate, since a future earnings lost projection is too simple a measure to accommodate the complex character of AIDS costs.

Lost earnings projections do not, for example, factor in the extraordinary toll of major talent that this epidemic is recording. Anyone who reads the collective summaries that occasionally appear cannot help but be impressed with the economic and creative significance of many of those afflicted.[10] Major figures in many fields have been infected; some are still well, some have died, others are fighting. In politics the list includes notables like Paul Gann, a leader in California Republican politics; Sheldon Andelson, regent of UCLA, whose Los Angeles home was referred to as the Western White House during the Kennedy years; Roy Cohn, the late Senator Joseph McCarthy's principal counsel on the Internal Security Subcommittee; Terry Dolan, master GOP fundraiser and founder of the National Conservative Political Action Committee. People in show business like Amanda Blake, the popular Miss Kitty of "Gunsmoke"; Rock Hudson; Liberace; William Bennett, the choreographer of "A Chorus Line"; and Larry Kramer, author and playwright. The noted fashion designers Perry Ellis and Roy Halston, as well as one of America's leading fine art photographers, Robert Mapplethorpe, have died. Actress and author Dorothy Mueller; Malcolm Forbes, publisher of *Forbes Magazine*; Methodist Bishop Finis Crutchfield of Texas; Dr. Tom Waddel, Olympic athlete; and France's Michel Foucault, one of the twentieth century's leading intellectuals, are also on the dread list.

In my hometown of San Antonio, a civic leader named "Hap" Veltman succumbed in 1989. He was one of the handful of local businessmen who, years ago, had the vision and drive to inspire downtown revitalization and historic preservation; everyone in San Antonio lives in a more beautiful city partly because of him. Every major city can now record similar names and cases. The costs of losing people of this calibre are staggering, ultimately incalculable. Even more melancholy is the understanding that in back of men and women who did have the opportunity to enhance our national culture is a generation of young men and women who will not have the time to enrich us.

As we move from the intangibles of personal loss, through estimated manpower and creativity losses, to tangible matters like payouts, it is clear that the AIDS epidemic involves enormous sums. The insurance industry projects a $37 billion-a-year payoff in the early 1990s and as much as $50 billion by 2000. Of course, any figure produced by the industry will be self-servingly on the generous side to justify the industry's desire to avoid insuring this health risk altogether. Even if the estimates are exaggerated by 50%, they still reflect very large amounts that must be pro-rated out to all surviving private policyholders and eventually to the entire society.

On the profit side of the ledger, HIV is rapidly generating a multibillion-

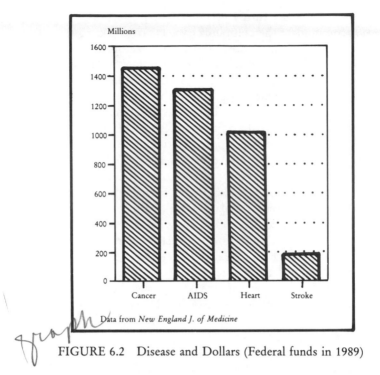

Data from *New England J. of Medicine*

FIGURE 6.2   Disease and Dollars (Federal funds in 1989)

dollar industry. The national government's aggregate AIDS-related expenditures went over the $2 billion mark in 1989 and will continue to rise. In addition, the combined states are spending over $500 million a year; this figure will also rise. These funds are funneled to scores of universities, medical research centers, and hundreds of community groups. Thousands of highly skilled researchers, laboratories, equipment companies, outreach workers, and the like are thus gainfully employed in an area that did not exist ten years ago.[11] In addition, an entirely new crop of AIDS-related companies reflecting hundreds of millions in capitalization have sprung up to produce and market everything from genetically engineered vaccines to safe-sex dolls.[12]

The market potential in all the aspects of AIDS stimulates the business oriented, including the con man, both here and abroad.[13] One of the corporations listed in a *Wall Street Journal* review of new AIDS-related businesses, Amnion Inc., estimated a $100 million per year market in just their area of blood recycling machines. Another firm estimates a $3 billion per year market in diagnostic tests within 10 years. The year 1988 experienced an international shortage (and price increase) in surgical rubber gloves and, after decades of languishing ashamedly in the pharmacist's drawer, the condom now proudly occupies its own display area in markets and drug-stores. In June 1990 the firm headed by Dr. Jonas Salk, developer of the polio vaccine, announced at the Sixth International Conference on AIDS that his group (The Immune Response Corporation) was in the testing stage of a promising therapeutic vaccine.[14] The market for an effective preventive and/or therapeutic vaccine staggers the imagination; every sexually active human being on Earth could potentially be inoculated, until the virus is no longer a serious threat to our species.[15] The bottom line is that the epidemic is a worldwide reality that national economies must confront in a variety of ways. Millions will die from AIDS, billions of dollars in public and private capital will be spent to combat it, and even more billions in new income will be generated by it.

HEALTH CARE COSTS

Direct health care costs are extremely difficult to estimate at this stage of the epidemic. The Skitovsy study cited earlier estimates that by 1991 hospital costs will have reached $8.5 billion annually, with PWAs occupying 1.2% of the available beds and accounting for 1.4% of the total personal health care expenditure.[16] Additional direct costs include hundreds of millions of dol-lars in testing, blood screening, research, and education. At the individual level it is estimated that the average lifetime cost of care (that is, lifetime remaining after diagnosis) will be between $60,000 and $70,000.[17] Adding the indirect costs of lost productivity to this produces an estimated overall cost that approaches $100 billion in 1991.

However, even these figures fail to convey the full impact of AIDS. They do not include any direct costs other than those calculated from the time of diagnosis until death, a period that has averaged (in the years 1985–1990) 13–18 months. But AIDS can have an incubation period of up to 11 years. During most of that period the individual ordinarily incurs no substantial medical expenses associated with the infection, although there can be some—costs of testing as well as medical and/or psychological consultation. After that, a mounting tide of bills can swamp the economy of the uninsured individual as he or she begins to encounter symptoms and illnesses that are debilitating, but short of the formal definition of AIDS. An example of the problem on the personal level can be drawn from the case of AZT. In August 1989 the Department of Health and Human Services, recognizing the benefits of early low-dosage use of AZT for non-AIDS diagnosed, asymptomatic seropositives, tripled the number (to 600,000) for whom AZT can be prescribed by physicians. For those who can afford it, the cost is now about $6500/annually at the standard 1200 mg/day dosage. It is hoped that new lower dosages (600 mg/day) will be as effective and lower the cost. Of course, these figures reflect the cost of the drug alone, not the additional cost of physician services in relation to diagnosis and prescription.[18] Regardless of dosage, however, the drug is still unavailable to the HIV+ unless he or she has private funds or insurance. After the individual is formally diagnosed with AIDS, he or she may obtain the drug under a state Medicaid program during the terminal stage of illness.[19] The total national cost of just this one medication, assuming all those who needed it had access, would be from $2 billion to $5 billion per year, depending on dosage. The manufacturer, Burroughs Wellcome, is sitting on an AIDS goldmine.

While high, it does not appear that the calculable health care costs of AIDS are out of line with those resulting from other serious traumas. The lifetime per-patient cost for persons suffering a major heart attack (mycardial infarction) is $66,837; for cancer of the digestive system, $47,542; for leukemia, $28,636; and for paraplegia from an auto accident, $68,700. The figure of $55 billion mentioned above as the value of lost productivity may seem high, but actually it is expected to be no more than 12% of the total figure in 1991. AIDS is costly and getting more expensive each day, but it is not so costly as to have structural impact on the American economic system. To put it another way, the American economy can absorb the impact of AIDS and, as a matter of fact, can afford and ought to allocate more funds for research, education, and treatment than it now does. This is not true for some Third World economies; AIDS has the potential of breaking their backs and pushing whole nations back 50 years in developmental time.[20]

The projection of costs leads inevitably to the question, who picks up the bill? In thinking about this, it is useful to apply the classic apportioning model of personal injury law. With regard to any injury (or illness), the cost can first of all be borne by the injured party. You have parked your car at the curb. Overnight a hitherto unsuspected subsurface sinkhole collapses, swallowing your car. You pay. Or, second, the one whose action led to the injury can be held liable for costs. You have parked your car. Your neighbor comes home late, suffers a stroke while driving, and sideswipes your car. He pays. Finally, the costs can be allocated among third parties who are strangers to the events leading to injury or ailment. One or both of you have purchased comprehensive insurance covering such unforeseen calamities. In that case, payment is assumed by all policyholders in the group to which you belong. The group can be privately defined, as with a Blue Cross policy, or publicly defined, as in Medicare or Medicaid. There are, of course, many permutations, combinations, and nuances in the actual design and administration of these alternatives, but at bottom there are only the basic three to work with. Stating the alternatives is easy, but nothing else in the field of tort or personal injury law is straightforward. Except in the simplest of cases, the equities of apportioning cost raise philosophic, jurisprudential, and legal problems that tax our finest minds. Indeed, the main thrust of modern practice has been legally to insist that everyone carry insurance so questions of individual apportionment do not rise at all; no-fault auto insurance and assigned risk pools are examples.

Applying this model to the costs of AIDS care leaves little room to doubt that the wisest course of public policy lies with the third alternative. Indeed, it is the only realistic one. It could be and has been argued that AIDS victims (except for pediatric and transfusion) should bear the cost of their illness since it was incurred in voluntary activities, sex or IV drug use. This is basically the position of the American far right, especially the evangelical, fundamentalist portion of it. Whatever quasi-religious arguments can be made, the real-world result would be that the afflicted would receive no care other than that which might come from private charity (presumably not the charity of the evangelical or fundamentalist). The suggestion that the cost be shared or borne by the "injurer" would lead to the same result. First, it would be difficult in most cases to establish the identity of the injuring party—who is the injurer in IV drug transmission? Second, even if identification were possible (as it is in some cases), the position generally leads to the shifting of costs to another sick and dying person who cannot pay his or her own bills. This is not to say that in some individual cases these positions might not make some sense. However, as a matter of public or general policy, they both lead to the same result, no treatment and no care. Assuming the American community evolves a compassionate response, then it must amortize over time and apportion over the entire population the costs of this disaster, just as it has done with the catastrophic costs associated with other aspects of being human, like aging, or injury from an earthquake.

While common sense appears to indicate a national insurance approach, this may not be a sufficient argument for the sorely tried taxpayer, who is asked to foot the bill for a seemingly endless list of late twentieth-century crises. What is the general taxpayer interest that justifies the expenditure of billions? The justification arises from the fact that we are all bound together, like it or not, in a hazardous urban life style. The policy of the state cannot eliminate the hazards and risks of this fact. However, it can alter and distribute the attendant costs in order to alleviate the burden, a catastrophic burden in the case of AIDS, to any single individual. For example, it permits, and in some cases mandates, the shifting of accident costs, incidental to industrial process, to the large group that consumes the product. It does not demand that the individual worker or employer shoulder the entire risk of producing the article the public wants, but which cannot be produced with total safety. When you purchase a car, part of the price reflects the cost of the inevitable worker injuries that will occur in its manufacture. When you drive it on the expressway you will, unknowingly, already have paid for the worker injuries and deaths incurred in the construction of it. You and the workers are bound together in an invisible community of interest. For different reasons, you both have a vital interest not only in the production process, but in the safety of that process. In addition, the state can pay costs directly out of general funds, which is another kind of apportionment by which the cost is spread through the entire taxpaying community. Examples of this approach would be the approximately one-half billion dollars in non-Medicaid disbursements from the state governments for AIDS. By 1991 it is expected that Federal matching Medicaid funds will add another $1.8 billion.

What is the community of interest that binds together the sick and the well? Why should the well be willing to assume, as third-party payers, the costs of those caught up in this epidemic or, indeed, any epidemic? First, we are and should feel bound together by the reality of our own frailty and vulnerability as unaided individuals. Any other posture is self-destructively arrogant. We need to remind ourselves of the unpleasant truth that such very expensive programs as are now funded, for example, to defray the high but life-giving costs of kidney dialysis might well be paralleled in a program that any of us could need in the future. To support and help the afflicted is to invest in our own future well-being. This is especially and poignantly true in the case of AIDS for the simple reason that, as pointed out in Chapter 2, HIV is *our* virus. We have no really good animal models to test vaccines and drugs. Consequently, the only authoritative source of information, which we all need for our protection, is that developed in testing and treatment protocols using fellow humans as volunteers. The quality of health care available to each of us is built squarely on the experience gained in caring for those who got sick before us.

In our search for treatments it is not possible to distinguish in principle between "nice" supportable afflictions and "unapproved" afflictions; the viral, bacterial, and fungal agents of our various ailments make no such distinctions. Only 40 years ago having cancer was unmentionable—cancer was a sin as well as a sickness. John Wayne and his studio feared, with good cause, that if the public knew of his bout with lung cancer, it would end his acting career; cancer, the "Big C," was the 1940s equivalent of leprosy. Similarly, former Congressman Coelho's childhood epilepsy was believed by his parents to be a divine punishment, and his church refused to accept him as a student for the priesthood.[21] One can only hope that at least a voting majority, if not all of us, have graduated from this level of stupidity.

Second, on another level each of us clearly shares a community interest in the quality of public health. Commencing with the Pure Food and Drug Act and Meat Inspection Act of 1906, we have manifested our concern through a host of statutory regulations and programs ranging from food-handling inspections to wide-ranging grants of power to track, control, or abate various infectious diseases. The Federal and state Public Health Services, which have played such a prominent role in educating us, owe their very existence to this social interest. The Centers for Disease Control and all our national and state regulations reflect the truth that, in a crowded urban civilization, the well-being of each of us is tied to the health of all of us. HIV is not the first, nor will it be the last dangerous virus to spread rapidly in our urban culture. Virologists are constantly tracking and trying to contain pestilential agents that break out of their home base, and more than one health care worker has died in the containment attempts. Indeed, epidemiologists are now recommending the establishment of international tracking stations, outposts that could give us fair warning that a breakout has occurred—the viral equivalent of our hurricane-tracking facilities.

There is no sensible, realistic option but to express our group interests with group techniques. The application of group insurance programs to cover AIDS is the only approach that makes sense. The group can be defined as a large cohort of employees in a single firm, or the entire population of the nation, whichever works best, but it is an exercise in futility to attempt to resolve a general problem with case-by-case individual decisions. The national $500 billion bailout of insolvent savings and loans associations is an example from outside the public health area; this failure of government to effectively regulate savings and loan management will cost each of us at least $5000 in taxes. What is the community of interest between the sick and the well in this epidemic? It is simple: the sick want to get well, and the well do not want to get sick, and in the end both are dependent upon coordinated group action to plan and fund the epidemic's containment as well as to subsidize the development of effective treatments and/or vaccine safeguards.

The epidemic has sharply underscored the fact that the United States, alone among major nations, has neither a unified, coherent health care insurance system, nor a method of rapid, effective drug testing and delivery—in spite of the fact that Americans spend more on illness than any other people. Medicare is a program limited to the elderly, who are largely unaffected by the epidemic, or those who have been "disabled" for two years. Medicaid for the poor is actually 50 different state programs, many of which lack benefits or access rules appropriate to a disease like AIDS. In Texas as in other states, for example, those who become eligible for Social Security disability automatically lose their national Medicaid entitlement. However, unlike other states, Texas does not substitute a state program for the lapsed national one. This means that there is a two-year hiatus of medical insurance coverage for the patient between the time of Medicaid's end and the triggering of Medicare. Most AIDS patients do not last that long; they die before satisfying state and national eligibility rules. As taxpayers who have helped fund these programs, they are defrauded by the rules.

Finally, about 35 million to 50 million Americans have no health insurance at all. Our nation accepted a basic responsibility for the health of its citizens only in the administration of President Lyndon Johnson, although there had been agitation for action as far back as the first term of President Franklin Roosevelt in 1932. We have moved slowly, hesitantly, and with a lack of efficiency, cost, and quality control that only a very rich nation could tolerate. Gradually, and partly as a result of the AIDS epidemic, major business and political leaders are recognizing this fact of our history, and speaking out for reform. In April 1989 Chrysler's Lee Iacocca suggested that "maybe we should go to school on the national health care systems in Europe and Japan and design one for ourselves."[22] More significantly, the American Medical Association is now proposing what is, in effect, a national health plan to restructure the U.S. system so that it would cover all Americans. The AMA's program is called Health Access America, and it represents a striking departure from the AMA's former stance of opposing anything smacking of "socialized medicine."[23] AIDS may be the proverbial straw that breaks the back of America's complacency and short-sightedness.

EMERGENCE OF NATIONAL POLICY

As has been said in this work many times, the HIV epidemic is a natural phenomenon obeying biological laws of mutation, transmission, and survival. So also is politics a natural phenomenon, a natural expression of our species. Politics is basically about the continuing struggle of all of us for a piece of the pie (which we now call the gross national product); it is about who gets what, where, and when. At its best, it is a governed and orderly competition that is geared to respond to tangible power as measured by aggregated capital and voting blocs. At its worst, it is war. But neither in peace nor in war does the political system respond to claims of compassion and humanity as readily as it does to claims of power. Like the virus, politics operates in accordance with many set rules—Machiavelli cataloged many of them in *The Prince*—and it would be foolish to expect these rules to be displaced because an epidemic entered the land.

The business of the politician, the art of governing, is that of compromising, conciliating, and finding accommodation for the various claims emerging from people's lives and dreams. The politician builds bridges among peoples and interests, does so within finite budgets and resources, and works in a twilight zone where the line between ethical and unethical conduct is sometimes hard to see. Queen Elizabeth I, a consummate royal politician, called her policy on church matters (the policy that served as the foundation for the Anglican/Episcopal church) the path of "The Golden Mediocritie." Somehow, that says it all. When the politicians fail, we resort to force. Epidemics are hard for politicians to cope with. Epidemics are about death and dying, about pain and suffering, and they are bad for business. They confound the political system. The politician cannot run "for" an epidemic or "against" it; both postures would be silly. Effectively coping with global catastrophes such as AIDS do call for truly great and courageous political leadership, something that is in short supply everywhere. The lack of it in America during the past few decades is one of many factors that have allowed both an epidemic and a drug culture to take firm root in the land.

Of course, some issues are more amenable to political resolution than others. It is one thing to construct a coalition over the design of the new city hall, quite another to do so when emotionally charged issues like slavery, abortion, drug use, death, or sex are involved. In these areas our treasured cultural mythologies and religious codes often conflict with real-world facts, making a reasonable decision difficult. Politicians quite rightly think of such issues as "no win" issues, and shy away if possible. For example, most heterosexuals firmly believe that homosexuality is unnatural and sinful. They have been taught this by the ministers of the Western church since the days of St. Paul. He denounced all pleasurable, nonprocreative sex whether heterosexual or homosexual, regarded women largely as creatures who lure God-fearing men into lust and sin, and taught that, on the whole, it would be best if the species gave up all sex in order to prepare for the Day of Judgment, which he believed was just around the corner. St. Augustine and St. Thomas Aquinas seconded and elaborated his views later on. Given such a heritage, it is no wonder that today it is difficult to discuss any sexual issue rationally in the political area.

An illustration of the impact of our sex-negative origins appears in the debate over whether to distribute condoms in prison. AIDS has become a leading cause of inmate death in all areas (like New York) with high seroprevalence levels. The major sexual mode of transmission is anal inter-course, which most prisoners do not regard as homosexual behavior in the closed, all-male prison environment. With few exceptions, those in charge of such matters have avoided the obvious policy.[24] To distribute condoms in an all-male prison community would be to admit openly and officially that illegal sex acts are taking place. It is certain that political opponents would make it appear that the decision-makers condoned such acts. Moreover, distribution of condoms would be tantamount to admitting that the police cannot enforce the law even in prison, and if not there, where? The upshot is that lives will continue to be sacrificed to the needs of myth maintenance and the political necessities of winning within America's sex-negative political arena.

Moreover, it is hard to make political capital out of an epidemic. This is not to say no one tries. In 1918 some charged that the Spanish flu, which killed over 500,000 Americans, had been deliberately introduced by German U-boats spraying the port of Boston with active virus. In the 1980s African political leaders denounced the West for the anti-black, neocolonial suggestion that the virus originated there, while some American political figures were looking for evidence that it was the product of Soviet genetic engineering. The Soviets, for their part, spread the rumor throughout Africa that the virus was another instrument of American biological warfare. The French, meanwhile, blamed American tourists, and we blamed Haitians and homosexuals. Oblivious to this nonsense, the virus continued to spread.

REAGAN AND AIDS

The first five years of American political reaction to the surfacing of AIDS was a compound of deprecation, derision, disbelief, and denial. Clearly the most important single variable determining political reaction was the early identification of AIDS with homosexual sex. Neither Walter Mondale nor Ronald Reagan, the presidential candidates, nor any official or party document made reference to AIDS in the campaigns of 1984 even though, by that time, public health experts and agencies were issuing alarms. It was largely Rock Hudson's highly publicized death in 1985 that forced national politics out of the AIDS closet to admit the danger and begin forming policy. President Reagan acknowledged the existence of AIDS only when his friend died a celebrity's death while a stunned world watched. By the time he did acknowledge the epidemic, 20,000 Americans had died.

The administration's response was slow and reluctant; public statements and administration policy indicated that a calculation had been made to the effect that those most affected were of little political consequence to the fortunes of the Republican party and, consequently, there was no need for vigorous action.[25] No agency of the Reagan administration made an official budget request relating to AIDS until the FY1985 proposals were sent to Congress. These came three years after the first alarms were sounded. In 1982 and 1983 Congress, acting on its own initiative, appropriated a total of about $34 million, and established the pattern of congressional, rather than presidential, leadership that persists to the present. Reagan's reluctance to address the issue ran counter to the strongly worded advice of the National Academy of Sciences and a virtually unanimous public health establishment.[26] The President's basic attitudes can best be inferred, perhaps, from the budgets he presented over the years of his administration (Table 6.1).

Only in his last, going-out-of-office set of proposals for FY1990 did his recommendations approximate the amounts called for within his own administration and, even then, the sum was no more than the cost of one nuclear submarine.[27]

TABLE 6.1   Request for AIDS Funding, 1983–1990 (in million of dollars)

FISCAL YEAR	PUBLIC HEALTH ESTABLISHMENT REQUEST	PRESIDENTIAL REQUEST	CONGRESSIONAL REQUEST
1983	—	—	5.5
1984	—	—	28.7
1985	59.9	39.8	61.4
1986	91.0	60.5	108.6
1987	196.0	126.4	244.3
1988	351.0	213.2	355.4
1989	(Consolidated)	766.4	951.0
1990	1600.0	1300.0	1200.0

Source: *National Journal*, August 30, 1986, p. 2046.

In response to growing criticism of his inaction, Reagan established a Presidential Commission on AIDS in 1987. The opening months of the commission's life were most unpromising, as the body was paralyzed by internal bickering; it was generally characterized as long on conservative politicians and short on AIDS experts. The first co-chairpersons resigned in disgust,[28] leading to the appointment of Admiral James D. Watkins (Ret.) as chairperson. Admiral Watkins turned the commission around dramatically. He proved to be another Surgeon General Koop. A conservative officer who was expected to remain quietly within Reagan policy guidelines, Watkins became an ardent and articulate spokesperson for vigorous Presidential leadership and national action. Faced with the realities of the epidemic, the Presidential Commission produced a report in June 1988 with 579 recommendations, many of which called for policies strongly opposed by representatives of the ideological right in the White House.[29] The Commission recommended the authorization of almost $2 billion more than the 1989 appropriation for AIDS and the related problem of drug abuse.[30] The outcome was that President Reagan declined to support his own Commission's recommendations. Dr. Donald Ian MacDonald, the President's spokesperson, explained that the "White House" felt that some of the Commission's central recommendations (for example, those calling for Federal laws to guarantee confidentiality of HIV test results or prohibit various forms of discrimination) would amount to rewarding "disapproved" behaviors.[31] Presumably, if someone faced social, employment, or legal problems due to disclosure of positive test results, it was only just deserts. The fact that lack of confidentiality would effectively undermine any national testing program was considered irrelevant to the main moral and political issue. Instead of supporting his Commission, President Reagan issued a policy paper in August 1988 that Washington quickly dubbed the "Reagan 10-Point Inaction Plan."[32]

PLAGUE OR EPIDEMIC?

During the 1985–1988 period AIDS-related political coalitions began to take shape, and they tended to polarize around the basic postures outlined in Chapter 1—that is, the nonjudgmental, epidemic position on the one hand, and the religiously judgmental, plague position on the other. Powerful spokespersons for both positions appeared in the national and state governments. Agency officials concerned with biomedical research, public health, and epidemic control were compelled to walk a political tightrope between them. Complicating matters at the national level was the fact that the Reagan administration was publicly and firmly committed to a tight money policy with regard to all nondefense domestic spending. The additional research and public health expenditures needed to fight the epidemic promised to "unbalance" the budget.

The leading national actors who emerged during this period representing the "epidemic" position were Surgeon General C. Everett Koop in the administration, and in the Congress Senators Edward Kennedy (D-Mass.) and Lowell P. Weicker, Jr. (R-Conn.) and Representative Henry A. Waxman (D-Cal.). The "plague" position was articulated in the administration by Secretary of Education Edward Bennett and in the Congress by Senator Jesse Helms (R-N.C.) and Representative William E. Dannemeyer (R-Cal.). It would be inaccurate to see the two blocks as matching a liberal-conservative or Democratic-Republican split. For example, Senator Orrin Hatch (R-Utah), a leading conservative, was and remains a strong backer of the public health approach, supporting the initiatives of his Democratic colleagues in the Senate. Likewise, the leading Reagan administration "epidemic" spokesperson, Surgeon General Koop, considered himself a social and political conservative. On the other hand, it is true that those coming from the "plague" perspective have tended to be mostly, but not entirely, conservative Republicans.[33] Back of each of these two groups of officials were loosely defined coalitions of social, religious, and economic interests which, for one reason or another, had and continue to have a stake in AIDS-related government policy.

The fundamental difference between the two positions stems from their reaction to the large number of homosexuals among the afflicted.[34] The plague position is essentially negative from the standpoint of government intervention. Federal money ought not be used for people whom Senator Helms, resurrecting Victorian terminology, refers to as "sodomites." Their sex practices are rejected by the American public and their affliction is a well-deserved punishment of God. His judgment on IV drug users is not noticeably more benign. Consistent with this approach, Senator Helms fought the authorization of funds to help AIDS patients purchase AZT, and Representative Dannemeyer called for "routine" mandatory testing without guarantees that the results would be legally confidential. Proponents of this stance in the administration and Congress have successfully resisted efforts to modify Medicaid access rules for the benefit of PWAs who were dying before qualifying.

On the other hand, significant expenditures for research on vaccines is accepted as a long-term investment in the health of the heterosexual community, although why the non-sinful should need such protection is not clear. Money for infected children is justified as appropriately Christian. Federally financed public education is admitted to be necessary, but campaigns must be decorous in language so as, to quote a leading Victorian, "not to bring a blush to fair maiden's cheek" or, more to the point in the 1990s, not to offend America's politically potent religious conservatives.[35] Secretary Bennett successfully insisted that public educational material emphasize sexual abstinence and undefined "family values" rather than condom use.[36] Nancy Reagan's now famous motto, "Just say no!", became the battle cry for both the "war on drugs" and the "war on AIDS."

These attitudes were frequently mirrored at the state level. For example, the 1989 Texas public health budget tried to ensure that not a penny would fall into the hands of community groups that may be "gay operated," even though such groups have been the agencies that have pioneered effective hospice programs and provided a large part of needed care to everyone regardless of mode of infection. Following Secretary Bennett's lead, the state also severely curtailed state distribution of condoms, a stupidity which is very apt to surface later in the form of an increased incidence of teen-age AIDS.[37] The Texas legislation required all educational materials to stress the illegality of homosexuality and drug usage and the virtues of abstinence. It also required the state Department of Health to trace sexual partners of infected individuals. However, few of these provisions were supported by the funding necessary to make them administrative realities. The legislative debate was more a public protestation of virtue ("We are all straight, Christian, non-drug users.") for the purpose of electioneering than an attempt to formulate sensible policy for the state that has the distinction of ranking 4th in number of cases, 8th in population seroprevalence level, and 37th in per capita AIDS expenditures.[38]

As noted in Chapter 1, this generally negative stance has deep roots in the American heritage. Senator Helms and Representative Dannemeyer forced many of their colleagues to risk political futures in order to vote for sensible

Federal programs to contain the epidemic. Every vote in favor of positive programs lent itself to being represented as a vote that was "soft" on "queers," junkies, and/or criminals. As Governor Dukakis can testify from his 1988 presidential campaign experience, being so labeled confers no advantage in American politics. It is testimony to more legislative courage that we are apt to give credit, that the "plague" position from 1987 has become increasingly a minority, rear-guard action unable to stop the emergence of a coherent national policy on AIDS.

The adherents of the "epidemic" position, on the other hand, argue that the citizenry's varied sexual dispositions and habits of substance abuse[39] are irrelevant to the battle, except as factors to be considered in designing specific and targeted public health strategies. The epidemic of HIV is and should be regarded as a menace to the entire nation, and national public health policy should not be affected by any individual's moral judgment regarding the behavior of those who have been or may become infected. It is pointed out that even where there is a very low probability of an individual's seroconverting, that person is nonetheless endangered by the AIDS-assisted resurgence of other diseases such as tuberculosis. After a decade of decline, TB began a comeback in 1986.[40] The epidemic position has been clearly articulated by conservatives like Surgeon General Koop and liberals like Senator Kennedy. It is the position which from 1988 set the tone (with a few exceptions) for national policy; its major legislative statements are the HOPE Act, the Health Omnibus Programs Extension Act of 1988, the national government's initial attempt at a coherent policy on AIDS,[41] and the Ryan White Act of 1990.

THE HOPE ACT AND NATIONAL POLICY

The first thing one senses in the Act is an undercurrent of urgency that was notably lacking in previous official statements. The second is that its broad divisions do recognize the various areas of policy relevant to a coherent approach to the epidemic. In summary terms and commencing October 1, 1988, the Congress authorized $400 million for three years of testing, $200 million for two years' support of home health care programs, $285 million to $300 million for three years of research (there are other portions of the Federal budget that support much additional research), $250 million to $300 million for three years of AIDS education, and $2 million to fund a new, permanent National AIDS Commission. The provisions of the Act can be conveniently grouped under eight policy headings:

Scientific/Medical Research. The single largest commitment of national policy up to 1988 had been to funding basic scientific research into the nature of the virus and medical research seeking effective vaccines, drugs, and treatments. The statute confirms previous priorities in the allocation of

AIDS funds. However, there is a new emphasis on expediting grants and evaluations—a response to the frequent complaint that such matters were unduly delayed in the national bureaucracy. A very important change is the statutory mandate to broaden the concept of "testing and evaluation" beyond the traditional laboratory-experimental model. Scientists are mandated to devise new protocols of evaluation that are quicker, even if less certain, than the classical ones. In this vein, the statute authorizes the establishment of AIDS-specialized research centers, clinical research review committees, NIH clinical evaluation units, and methods of evaluating treatments not approved by the government. These provisions constitute a partial victory for those involved in the clinical treatment of PWAs over laboratory scientists who generally have not recognized the legitimacy of research findings unless supported by strict protocols. Provision is also made for the continuation of basic genetic research into the structure and operation of the virus as well as social science research programs connected to the impact and control of the epidemic. At the global level, Congress authorized support of vaccine research in other countries and the programs of international agencies such as the World Health Organization and the Pan American Health Organization.

Professional Information and Education. A major problem confronting those working professionally has been the explosion of research activities and information. There is so much now available that the problem is one of access, of simply knowing that a particular study has been done and where to find it. Congress addressed this and similar problems by authorizing two national data banks, one for basic AIDS research and another for clinical trials and treatments. With such computerized facilities it becomes possible to disseminate information rapidly, avoiding duplication of effort. It also authorized special educational programs to overcome both professional and lay ignorance of the uses and risks of transfusion as well as blood donation. To provide more adequate data on the behavior and spread of HIV in various groups, Congress authorized the establishment of epidemiological and mortality rate data bases as well as a national seroprevalence survey. The latter has helped launch possibly the most politically sensitive survey the national government has ever tried to conduct, the *National Household Seroprevalence Survey*, which asks citizens to undergo anonymous blood tests and answer intimate questions about their sexual behavior.[42]

Direct PWA Care. A segment (about 13%) of the overall budget is dedicated to direct care through grants for home and community care services, subsidized AZT, the development of model care protocols, and community-based evaluation of experimental therapies. The allocation for direct care is so modest that it gives credence to speculation that Reagan made an unadmitted decision to withhold all but token aid to the one million already infected, a decision that appears to receive quiet but continued support from both the epidemic and plague coalitions.[43] This position has been incorrectly referred to as a triage decision. But this is inaccurate. Triage is the morally justifiable division of battlefield casualties into three groups: (1) those who will die whether or not care is given, (2) those who will live whether or not care is given, and (3) those who require care to survive. Medicine and attention under battlefield conditions, where all resources are in short supply, are reserved for the third group. But no such conditions existed in the United States. We were at peace and had abundant resources; there was and there is no morally justifiable reason for the decision to withhold care and write off the infected. It remains a tragic departure from standard American policy in such matters. As a nation we have long since made the basic decision that we should strongly support programs for medically managing, prolonging, and generally improving the quality of life remaining for those living with catastrophic afflictions; kidney dialysis centers and aid for various handicaps come to mind. I believe that we will, one day, classify this position as another of the sorrier moral lapses of American politics and list it with such events as the imprisonment of Japanese-Americans during World War II, and the slaughter of native Americans.

Testing and Counseling. Provision is made for grants to states that operate HIV testing and counseling programs. The Federal guideline calls for the testing to be anonymous and insists that there be counseling provided as an integral part of the testing program.

General Public Education. Bloc grants-in-aid to the states are provided to encourage the development of general as well as specially targeted educational programs. Special target programs might be directed toward ethnic minorities, health care or public safety workers, or any group the unique characteristics of which call for special approaches. In addition, the Act calls for the establishment of a national AIDS information clearinghouse and a 24-hour toll-free hotline (1-800-458-5231).

Professional Training. Funds are provided for incentive subsidies and loans to encourage students to train in the specialized subfields of AIDS treatment and research as well as continuing education coursework for those already in the profession.[44]

Felons. State grants-in-aid are provided to encourage the establishment of HIV testing of sex offenders and IV drug users.

Organizational. Congress mandated the establishment of an Office of AIDS Research directly under the Director of the National Institute of

Health, emphasizing the high priority Congress placed on this work. Furthermore, Congress established a National AIDS Commission of 15 members (five appointees each from the President, the Senate, and the House) to "promote the development of a national consensus on AIDS policy, and make recommendations regarding such policy."

The policy expressed in the Act of 1988 was strongly oriented toward research and preventive education but was deficient in addressing the plight of those already afflicted. Further, since Congress had already appropriated its FY1989 AIDS-related money prior to the passage of the HOPE Act, the funding of the Act's provisions had to await 1990 hearings and 1991 implementation.[45] Some of this deficiency was dealt with in the Americans with Disabilities Act of 1990, which extended the antidiscrimination provisions of three previous Federal statutes to those who, by the act's definition, are "disabled"—a category that includes PWAs.[46] The Act makes it illegal for businesses employing more than 25 persons to discriminate against people with disabilities in hiring and/or firing and arms the disabled with Federal remedies to fight discrimination in housing and places of public accommodation like restaurants, theaters, and hotels.[47] The language of the statute has still to receive definitive court interpretation, and many questions remain. For example, it does not prohibit discriminatory treatment of the "ill," only the "disabled," and even in that context prohibits only the application of a general rule of discrimination to all disabled. An example of a general rule in operation could be seen in the uniform exclusion of PWAs from all San Antonio nursing homes. In 1988 the president of the San Antonio AIDS Foundation, a colorful and redoubtable man named Papa Bear, tried to get a 74-year-old lady with AIDS admitted to a nursing home; they all refused her. The Foundation then filed a complaint with the Office of Civil Rights of the Federal Department of Health and Human Services. Two years later (long after the lady had died) that office ruled the nursing homes in violation of Federal antidiscrimination regulations. If they fail to bring their admission policies into line with Federal regulations they will be denied Medicare and Medicaid funding.[48] Employers and landlords can still discriminate if they can justify their action with the facts of an individual case. The difficulty of justification will, of course, depend upon the general attitudes of the presiding arbitrator or judge.[49] President Reagan opposed the passage of the Disabilities Bill, but candidate Bush pledged to support it, and President Bush signed it into law.

Finally, in 1990 a new attitude emerged in Washington regarding the proper official position on AIDS; the "epidemic" view of AIDS became the foundation for a major piece of legislation. In early 1990 an AIDS disaster relief bill was introduced by Senators Kennedy and Hatch with 19 others. A modified version of this passed both Houses of Congress on August 4 and was sent to the President for signature. The Ryan White Comprehensive AIDS Resources Act (named after the Indiana teenager whose AIDS story and death captured the nation's sympathy) establishes as a matter of public policy that AIDS is to be conceived of and dealt with as the natural disaster it is. The Act authorizes broad assistance to the communities that have been hardest hit by the epidemic. It applies to communities with more than 2000 cases or an incidence of 25 cases per 100,000 population; in 1990 this included 16 American cities: Atlanta, Boston, Chicago, Dallas, Ft. Lauderdale, Houston, Jersey City, Los Angeles, Miami, New York, Newark, Philadelphia, San Diego, San Francisco, San Juan, and the nation's capital, Washington, D.C.

The Ryan White Act authorizes $4.5 billion over the next five years, including $882 million (FY 1991) for emergency aid to hospitals, state programs, and special pediatric care.[50] To qualify for Federal grants-in-aid the states must provide, at minimum, HIV blood testing with pre- and post-test counseling, further testing in the case of positive results to determine the extent of immune system impairment, and appropriate therapeutic measures, referrals, and medical evaluations of seropositive individuals. These provisions may be the beginning of a national testing program. The Act encourages the organization of consortia of agencies, both public and private, to pool resources to provide a care system which, in its totality, would cover all needed services from educational outreach programs to terminal care. Other provisions authorize special studies of HIV's movement into rural areas, programs to ensure the safety of the blood supply, and a partner notification study. The Act does permit fees to be charged for various services if the individual or family is above the poverty line ($5980 annual income per person in 1989). However, the fees are statutorily pegged as a percentage of income (5–10%) at various levels, and, further, the Act specifically provides that, in the last analysis, services will be provided without regard to ability to pay, or current or past health condition.

The act represents a major victory for those of the "epidemic" persuasion. As a matter of Federal policy, AIDS is viewed as a natural and national disaster. However, it should be kept in mind that the exceedingly complex legislative-executive appropriations process still offers many opportunities for those of the opposition "plague" mindset to lesson the impact of the Ryan White Act. I am reminded of the fact that Congress authorized the Prison Testing Act (PL 100–607) in 1988, but has not yet completely implemented it.

One of the more interesting requirements of the Act is that most of the funds to be allocated are to flow directly from Washington to "the top elected official in the metropolitan area who administers the public health

agency serving the largest number of individuals with AIDS in the area." [51]
There are several political implications of this directive. First, the Ryan
White provisions, in bypassing the central state health agencies, are intended
to produce more rapid and effective results at the municipal level where the
sick reside.[52] State health agencies, reflecting state legislative attitudes, have
sometimes not been overly responsive to the needs of PWAs. Second, the
budget that will be available to the municipal officer, plus the Act's emphasis
on the establishment of consortia (coordinated by the municipal officer), will
necessarily shift the locus of control over local AIDS programs and services
from private, volunteer AIDS service organizations to public health bureaucracies. Given the costs and complexities involved in effectively containing
AIDS, a government takeover is necessary and unavoidable. But for one like
myself, who has been involved in helping my local ASO, the San Antonio
AIDS Foundation, there is a sadness in watching the displacement of private
caring and initiative, and the development of still another government
program wherein an individual, in this case a very sick person, inevitably
becomes just another case number.

PROBLEMS OF NATIONAL POLICY

In confronting the bubonic plague in San Francisco and New York at the
turn of the century, the evolving U.S. Public Health Service (then called the
Marine Health Service) employed two techniques that were to become the
standard operating approach to epidemic control, namely quarantine and
sanitation. Other techniques were added as the service became more comprehensive and sophisticated, such as contact tracing of venereal or pneumonic disease carriers, public education, data gathering, and now epidemic
SWAT teams operating domestically and internationally. But one surprising
oversight, in a nation that prides itself on the sophistication of its internal
information system, is the lack of a uniform, national epidemic data collection and surveillance system. The Federal Centers for Disease Control
receives state-collected data on a number of diseases, which are reported in
the *Morbidity and Mortality Weekly Reports*. Many of these reportable
diseases can provide the biologic basis for an epidemic, but there is no
national surveillance system in place that can sound a warning. Had there
been a tracking system in place during the 1970s our response might have
come much earlier and been less political and more effective. In May 1989
the Council of State and Territorial Epidemiologists urged the creation of
such a system.[53] AIDS is not the first, nor will it be the last, epidemic faced
by America. There will be others produced by existing or mutant viruses.
Without an early warning system we are like chickens in a coop, with no
way of knowing the fox is coming.

A related problem has to do with the accuracy and timeliness of the data we need to track biological killers. Currently the national reporting system is dependent upon the efficiency of state health departments, which rely, in turn, upon accurate reporting from physicians, coroners, hospitals, and other local agents. Some states do a good job, some do not. But even among the most conscientious, the methods and categories of collection vary widely, so that the data coming from different states are not necessarily comparable, a fact that distorts the national picture. It seems incredible, but it is nonetheless true, that it is difficult to get an accurate picture of the problems infecting our body politic. In the field of AIDS, for example, a major obstacle to the collection of data has stemmed from the stigma associated with the disease. Because AIDS is seen by so many as a sickness that results from sin, there has been significant underreporting of the disease during treatment and as a cause of death.[54] Patients and relatives prevail upon those responsible for reporting the data to conceal the truth.

From the standpoint of national policy, both problems place additional strains on the Federal organization of the union. Clearly the agents of viral and/or bacterial death have no concern for the legal and political refinements of national-state relations. State boundaries are our invention, not nature's. An epidemic with national catastrophic potential, like a major depression, is a national problem and must be confronted with a unified national policy. The epidemic raises in an acute way the question of whether we can continue the luxury of dealing with health problems in a piecemeal way, state by state and program by program. By 1989 the 50 states and the District of Columbia had created a confusing patchwork of over 170 different laws involving the many aspects of HIV infection.[55] As surely as the Great Depression forced major changes in the relationship of the government to the economy, AIDS will push us toward a unified national health program including surveillance, insurance, regulation, drug development, professional certification, care, and funding.

HIV is also forcing a reappraisal of the traditional methods of coping with disease transmission. Quarantine of those infected, as a technique, is almost as old as epidemics themselves but seems completely inappropriate to AIDS. The purpose of a quarantine is to contain the epidemic agent within limited physical boundaries. Entire cities (especially harbor cities) were sealed off in an effort to contain the spread of the bubonic plague, cholera, and yellow fever, and vessels from epidemic areas were routinely held at anchor for 40 days. Such measures made sense for diseases like the bubonic plague, which were very easily transmitted, burned themselves out within a limited time, and presented readily identifiable symptoms.

But HIV infection is not such a disease. Unlike tuberculosis, for example, is it not transmissible by someone sneezing in the elevator or by a friendly social kiss. It requires participation in complex and intimate behavior, behavior we are not likely to abandon. Both sex and substance abuse of various kinds (drugs, liquor, pills) will be with us, I suspect, as long as death and taxes. And not until the final years of a long process, when terminal AIDS sets in, does it reveal itself publicly.

Moreover, effective quarantine, as a public health measure, implies several nationally administered tests of the entire population within a reasonably short time.[56] It also implies rapid and accurate test protocols. However, the evidence increasingly indicates that our most widely used tests have very serious limitations, not the least of which is a possible 18-month lapse between the time of infection and the appearance of test reaction.[57] Quite apart from the administrative problems and astronomical costs[58] of such an endeavor, it would encounter major legal and practical difficulties. How could the legitimate objections of various religious groups, such as Christian Scientists, to such a procedure be surmounted?

Finally, the results of such a survey could be rapidly undermined by international population movement unless America were to seal its borders. Along with 29 other nations,[59] the United States has instituted HIV+ related restrictions on travel into or through the United States, but their major impact so far has been to inspire boycotts of the Sixth International Conference on AIDS (San Francisco, June 1990) and a meeting of the World Federation of Hemophilia (August 1990, Washington, DC)[60] and to cause sponsors to start looking for a location other than the United States (Boston) for the next international gathering. In January 1991, The Secretary of Health and Human Services, Dr. Louis Sullivan, lifted the controversial ban. The dimensions of international population movement today make an effective self-imposed quarantine impossible. Each year there are an estimated 100 million travelers crossing borders by air transport alone, and possibly a billion if land crossings (legal and illegal) are added. Isolation from contamination either from within or without is no longer possible. Furthermore, to quarantine a person who tests HIV+ for perhaps a decade is inhumane. To do so would transmute a blood test result into an irrebuttable criminal charge with a life sentence. Such a process could not survive challenges under the due process, unreasonable searches and seizure, self-incrimination, and/or cruel and unusual punishment clauses of the U.S. Constitution.[61] Finally, no one in their right mind would volunteer to be tested under such circumstances. A national screening would have to be mandatory, with all the police-state implications of such an approach.

Similarly, the traditional contact tracing and sanitation techniques are much more limited in their efficacy within the AIDS context. The invasion of constitutionally protected privacy involved in tracing an infected person's sexual contacts is clearly justified in the case of, say, gonorrhea, by the fact that the infected person, once found, can be cured and the chain of transmission broken. Until very recently, however, HIV contact tracing could only serve more limited purposes. It could be important for gathering better epidemiological data, and the contact could enable social workers to warn a possibly infected person to practice safer sex lest he or she further transmit the deadly virus. However, the value society receives by an individually targeted safer sex warning, or by better data, has to be weighed against not only the very high cost of contact tracing, but also against the invasion of privacy entailed. Instead of a clear answer, we have cost-benefit analysis. On the other hand, today the evidence mounts that early intervention with low-dose AZT treatment may slow the progression to AIDS. Therefore, contact tracing could be the first step in treatment, but only if the national government makes available low-dose AZT for those who are found, through tracing, to have been infected. What would be the point otherwise?

Sanitation is, of course, an attempt to eliminate those conditions that facilitate the survival and transmission of the infectious agent. The great historical clean-ups easily come to mind: spraying or draining stagnant water areas to kill mosquito larva (yellow fever, malaria), eliminating easy access to rodent food supply and nesting areas (bubonic plague), ensuring that sewage does not drain into water supplies (cholera), and the establishment of government inspection programs for food processing, distribution, and preparation (food poisoning, from botulism to salmonella). However, the breeding ground of HIV is wherever humans can have sex or shoot drugs, which is everywhere, and the practices that must be abated are the most hidden, intimate, and resistant to change in our entire portfolio of human behaviors. The only obvious environmental targets are the various sex emporia that cater to people looking for transient, anonymous sexual encounters. The most famous operation along these lines was the controversial closing of San Francisco's gay baths, but San Francisco's lead was not necessarily followed elsewhere, and the idea was never applied to straight sex clubs. America may be worried about the AIDS epidemic, but not so much as to seriously attack our enormous sex industry or consistently police our favorite highways and byways of assignation.

Testing and contact tracing both raise the knotty problem of confidentiality which, in turn, is related to HIV+ counseling. This issue is one that separates the "plague" from the "epidemic" factions, and is one poorly understood by the general public. Almost everyone admits that testing must be anonymous in a disease with so many stigma-derived implications that the mere fact of having been tested, if known, may lead to discrimination. No one would volunteer for testing otherwise. However, the epidemic and plague groups part company when a seropositive result is obtained. How confidential should the results be? Positive test results have been used to deny military and other employment opportunities, deny or cancel insurance, close access to the ability to practice professions from teaching to medicine, and bar or delay entrance to the United States.[62]

The plague position runs from the extreme of insistence that the names of infected individuals ought to be publicly known, to a position that legal duties ought to be imposed on those who know of positive test results (like physicians) to notify those who have a "need to know"—spouses, health care workers, insurance companies, employers, and the like. The epidemic position runs from the extreme that only the testee has a right to know the result and has complete control over subsequent notification to others, to a position that those who know of positive test results have a duty to make a good faith effort to ensure that those who might be endangered (like sexual partners) be informed. There is no neat answer. It seems unconscionable for a physician not to ensure that sexual partners of an HIV+ be notified; on the other hand, to insist upon notification violates the essential privacy of doctor-patient relationships. The situation is analogous to that faced by psychiatrists, priests, and other counselors when they come into possession of information that clearly bears upon the safety of innocent third parties. You're damned if you do and damned if you don't.

The Ryan White Act, Title III requires the states (as a condition of receiving Federal money) to maintain confidentiality of information covering receipt of preventive or therapeutic health services, prohibits involuntary or unauthorized HIV testing, and mandates the availability of anonymous testing procedures. But the ambiguities inherent in this area, the horns of our private and public dilemma, show up in the ambiguous proviso that the Act's requirements be administered "in a manner not inconsistent with any applicable local, state or federal law," as well as provisions requiring state public health officers to trace and notify the partners of seropositive individuals.[63]

The nation, in the process of living with AIDS, is working out resolutions to many of these problems without coming to grips clearly with the principles involved. We are muddling through.[64] Given the numbers involved, general quarantine of all seropositive men, women, and children is administratively impossible whatever might be thought of its desirability, and, at the other end of the scale, even the least compromising civil rights advocates are backing away from the protection of those who deliberately ignore the safety of others.

However, issues of testing, confidentiality, and tracing still plague our public debate and conscience. No one denies that effective counseling must be tied to testing, especially for those who receive a positive result. But there are many arguments as to how aggressive testing should be and how available the test results should be. Stephen Joseph, the Commissioner of

Health for New York City, speaking to the Fifth International Conference on AIDS, predicted much more extensive, and possibly mandatory, government programs of testing, tracing, and quarantine as the epidemic picks up speed in America.[65] Aggressive, even mandatory, testing and tracing do make some sense, *but only if they are securely tied to a national entitlement to treatment and antidiscrimination protection.* Otherwise these public health techniques could easily degenerate into an insidious form of trial and punishment.[66] Finally, the issue of confidentiality is gradually becoming mooted by the simple fact that so many public and private agencies are now requiring an HIV test that the facts are becoming available, if not completely public domain.[67] In my experience at the San Antonio AIDS Foundation, it has frequently been the seropositive individual him or herself who has been the source of information. It is hard not to talk about something so traumatic with one's friends, and, once announced, the information circulates like all bad news, widely and quickly. As the nation moves into the 1990s the issue will not be how to protect against breaches of confidentiality, but how to protect against the employment, insurance, housing, education, health care, and other forms of discrimination that may follow.

However, to admit all these limitations and reservations does not dispose of the genuine social, legal, and public health problems associated with "AIDS assault," that is, knowingly transmitting or attempting to transmit the virus. There are many cases on record. In December 1990 San Antonio's police started searching for a 31-year-old parolee who was suspected of having deliberately infected a number of women. According to the testimony of one of his former companions, he wooed her with a story that he was dying of leukemia and wanted to father a child to carry on the family name. Later he told her that he had AIDS and had vowed to take as many people with him as possible before he died.[68] Can the law of homicide be altered to incorporate a virus as the lethal weapon, or, conversely, could one's infection by another in a voluntary sexual encounter become a possible defense in a retributory homicide? Every major police department and AIDS counseling agency now knows of infected male and female prostitutes who are aware of their infection but regard it as an unavoidable risk of the profession. Can an infected person who continues sexual activity be placed in custody (quarantined) to protect the rest of us from being harmed both by our own folly and his/her unwillingness to desist? Are we prepared to give a cooperative prostitute or hustler something like unemployment benefits if he/she ceases operation? If not, can we really believe that the individual will stop?

Our current public policy and legal codes have no good answers for the new crop of AIDS problems. The Ryan White Act, Title III requires the states to assure the federal government that their criminal laws are adequate to prosecute an HIV+ individual who, knowing his or her status, donates blood, semen, or breast milk with the specific intention of infecting others, or engages in sex or shares hypodermic needles with that intention.[69] As can be seen from this provision, the response of the Congress to the need for imaginative and innovative lawmaking was to pass the buck to the states.

AIDS is clearly the kind of illness which, at the epidemic level, affects every aspect of our existence—our art, our economy, our religious faith, our politics and law, and above all our very lives. What is the source of this extraordinarily pervasive influence? After all, there are many other catastrophic and incurable illnesses. Why is it that AIDS almost immediately distinguished itself as something apart, something much darker, more threatening than Alzheimer's disease, lung cancer, Lupus, the vicious Ebola fever, and many terminal illnesses? Some commentators have pointed to its impact on the younger, more productive age group; but, in truth, this is the same age group that is most affected by death by industrial accident, by falling, and by auto accident. How about the numbers involved? Actually AIDS has a long way to go to catch up with just one worldwide bout with the flu back in 1918. Is it due to the fact that sex is a transmission route? I think not. Syphilis was epidemic in Europe for two centuries and is reaching epidemic levels in contemporary America without causing the consternation of AIDS. But this is the first *fatal* disease that, among other ways, can be transmitted sexually. In a sense this is true, but sex has always been a deadly game, and we have not been deterred. As part of a campaign to promote condom use, people working in AIDS education came up with a wonderful poster with the caption, "I love you dear, but not enough to die for." It is a great slogan and should be persuasive. But the truth is that if we are genuinely caught in the throes of passion, we do not think of death. Caution is the first casualty of love. Every AIDS counselor talking to a recent seroconverter, and inquiring about whether the person practiced safer sex, has seen the sad shake of the head, the puzzled expression, and heard the statement, "I couldn't insist, I was in love."

There are many more explanations that have been offered to justify the special status AIDS has so rapidly achieved among the diseases rampant on this globe, but none really satisfy. I believe the explanation must be that we all realize on some gut, intuitive level that AIDS is the first, and possibly not the last, of a new series of diseases that will challenge the very existence of our species, something no other life form has been able to do until now. The afflictions may not necessarily be new in the biologic sense, although some may be. Rather, they are new in the sense that, given the nature of twenty-first century life, we are newly vulnerable to them. One does not need to be a virologist to understand that a virus that attacks the very walls that nature, over millions of years, has erected to protect us, is a challenge like none other. The human immunodeficiency virus, in enlisting our very immune system to destroy us, represents the most formidable natural challenge ever mounted to the existence of our species. This is what puts AIDS in a class by itself. We are not fighting for a few more years, or a buoyant feeling of energy and good health, we are fighting for our very lives. And for all we know, the viral strategy may be a winning one.

Notes

1. President Reagan's physician, Brig. Gen. John Hutton (now commander of Madigan Army Medical Center, Ft. Lewis, Washington, D.C.) stated that the former President thought of AIDS as something like measles, which would go away. Not until his friend Rock Hudson died of AIDS in 1985 did the President ask for an expert briefing on the epidemic. In other words, none of the warnings from university and government public health experts penetrated the phalanx of aides and advisers who controlled access to the Oval Office. See interview and article, *San Antonio Express-News*, September 1, 1989, p. 1.
2. Paul Monette expresses this reaction at the personal level in his moving account, *Borrowed Time: An AIDS Memoir* (New York: Avon Books, 1988).
3. An example would be the defense of the Gay bathhouses in San Francisco. See Randy Shilts, *And the Band Played On*.
4. The Sydney Dance Company's electrifying production of *After Venice*, based on Thomas Mann's *Death in Venice*. It toured the United States in 1989. Larry Kramer's hit Broadway show, *The Normal Heart* (New York: New American Library, 1985); his memoirs, *Reports from the Holocaust: The Making of an AIDS Activist* (New York: St. Martin's Press, 1989); and the play by William Hoffman, *As Is* (New York: Putnam and Sons, 1988). Christopher Davis' novel, *The Valley of the Shadow* (New York: St. Martin's Press, 1988); David Feinberg's *Eighty-Sixed* (New York: Viking/Penguin, 1989); and Paul Monette's *Borrowed Time: An AIDS Memoir* (San Diego, CA: Harcourt, Brace & Jovanovich, 1988); as well as his volume of poetry, *Love Alone: Eighteen Elegies for Rog* (New York: St. Martin's Press); and George Whitmore's *Someone Was Here: Profiles in the AIDS Epidemic* (New York: New American Library, 1987); Alice Hoffman's *At Risk* (New York: Putnam, 1988); Adam Mars-Jones and Edmund White, *The Darker Proof: Stories from a Crisis* (New York: New American Library, 1988); and John Preston, *Personal Dispatches: Writers Confront AIDS* (New York: St. Martin's Press, 1989). Also, Michael Klein (ed.), *Poets for Life: Seventy-Six Poets Respond to AIDS* (Glendale, CA: Crown, 1989); Billy Howard, *Epitaphs for the Living: Words and Images in the Times of AIDS* (Dallas, TX: Southern Methodist University Press, 1989); Andrew Holleran, *Ground Zero: Collected Essays* (New York: Morrow, 1988); and the poignant *Screaming Room* (New York: Avon Books, 1986) by Barbara Peabody, a mother. Across the nation there have been many art shows and photography exhibits focusing on AIDS, both as fundraisers and as expressions of the grief of those in the arts community.
5. For information about the ongoing AIDS Memorial write: Names Project

Foundation, P.O. Box 14573, San Francisco, CA 94114 (415-863-5511). The idea for the quilt came from Cleve Jones of San Francisco, one of the founders of the San Francisco AIDS Foundation. The Names Quilt now weighs over 16 tons, requires five miles of walkways among the panels, and has 60 miles of seams. The original showing in Washington, D.C., required a display space equivalent to two football fields on the Mall. It was for the last time fully displayed in October 1989 on the Mall in Washington. Now the entire quilt is too large, and will only be seen in sections. See also the excellent photo essay on this memorial, Cindy Rushkin, *The Quilt: Stories from the NAMES Project* (New York: Pocket Books, Simon & Schuster, 1988).

6. See the lengthy and excellent article, Donald I. Abrams, Jeannee Parker Martin, and Kenneth W. Unger, "Psychosocial Aspects of Terminal AIDS," *Patient Care*, November 30, 1989, p. 41.

7. A modern parallel is found in the story of a family unable to "bury" their kidnapped and murdered daughter because of the interminable legal processing of the killer. "For the Survivors, the Mourning that Never Ends," *New York Times*, National, March 2, 1989, p. 43.

8. Michel de Montaigne, *The Essays*, Chap. 22 (George Ives, trans.) (New York: Heritage Press, 1946).

9. Anne Skitovsky, "Estimates of the Direct and Indirect Costs of AIDS in the United States," in Alan F. Fleming *et al.* (eds.), *The Global Impact of AIDS*, Chap. 17 (New York: Alan R. Liss, 1988). This overall cost includes two variables: (1) morbidity-cost = wages lost due to illness or disability, and (2) mortality-cost = present value of future earnings lost from premature death. The mortality-cost component accounts for 94% of the total. In 1991 AIDS will account for 12% of the total indirect costs stemming from illness and premature death.

10. See *Newsweek*, August 1987.

11. See Ron Winslow, "US Spending on AIDS Research and Prevention Reaches Level of Outlays on Other Major Diseases," *Wall Street Journal*, June 15, 1989, p. B4.

12. See "The New Crop of AIDS-Related Companies," *Wall Street Journal*, September 1987. The *Journal* lists: Amnion Inc.; Applied Biotechnology, Inc.; Athena Neurosciences, Inc.; Biopure Corp.; British Biotechnology, Ltd.; Candace Pert Foundation; DSW Laboratories; Gensia; IDEC, Inc.; Immune Response Corp. (this is headed by Dr. Jonas Salk); MicroGeneSys, Inc.; Mikromed Screening, Inc.; Murex Corp.; Quidel Corp.; Tanox Corp.; United Biomedical, Inc.; and Viro Research Laboratories, Inc. All of these were formed between 1985 and 1988. There are, of course, many more now.

13. See Kathryn Graven, "Japanese Join World Push to Cure AIDS," *Wall Street Journal*, November 10, 1988, p. B4. On illegitimate operations see *Info-AIDS Mailer* (University BITNET Computer Information Network), August 23, 1989. One recent con game based in Houston, Texas even advertised its operation in the "Business Opportunities" classified section of the *San Francisco Chronicle* claiming, without authorization, that its venture had the sponsorship of singer Pat Boone (who is the Honorary National Chairman of the AIDS Foundation for Children). This "business opportunity" involved the use of the Spiral Wells coin collection devices that have appeared in various shopping malls. See *San Francisco Chronicle*, Herb Caen's column, August 12, 1989.

14. Notice in *San Antonio Express-News*, June 8, 1989.
15. There is a parallel in the global campaign to eradicate poliomyelitis. See "Progress toward Eradicating Poliomyelitis from the Americas," *Health InfoCom Network News*, August 30, 1989, p. 14.
16. Skitovsky, "Estimates," Chap. 17. The burden will be spread very unevenly, due to the concentration of cases in the major metropolitan areas. While America has a surplus of hospital beds, the facilities in places like New York will be severely strained. The estimate is that PWAs will occupy 25% of the city's beds. It may be that we will have to distribute the burden of care over the nation's hospital system by moving some patients to where the beds are, even though that takes them away from relatives, friends, and other needed support. Another possibility is the subsidized development of a hospice network that can provide adequate care short of the hospital standard.
17. Skitovsky, "Estimates," p. 139.
18. In September 1989 Burroughs Wellcome Co. cut the price of AZT by 20%. The company's high pricing of the drug had been a subject of considerable and increasingly heated protests by groups representing seropositives. See *New York Times*, September 19, 1989, p. 1.
19. In a classic ploy, little understood by the general public, Congress for FY1989 *authorized* but did not *appropriate* $15 million to assist patients who did not have the personal wealth to buy AZT. Similarly, it authorized but did not appropriate $30 million for FY1990. What this means is that *if* the administrator can find the money, *then* he can spend it. Practically speaking, he can "find" it only by reallocating money within his approved budget or, more simply, he can transfer funds from cancer, muscular dystrophy, or whatever, to AIDS. Congress forces him to choose between the frying pan and the fire. It appears to the public that Congress is really providing new money for AIDS; it is not.
20. See the fine series of four articles by Eric Ekholm with John Tierney, "AIDS in Africa," which commenced in the *New York Times*, September 16, 1990.
21. *Congressional Quarterly*, August 8, 1989.
22. "Biting the Insurance Bullet: As Health Care Costs Rise, CEO's Warm to National Plan," *Newsweek*, August 28, 1989, p. 46.
23. For summaries of the AMA's plan as well as some others see the official bulletin of the AMA, *American Medical News*, March 16, 1990.
24. Theodore M. Hammett, National Institute of Justice, *1988 Update: AIDS in Correctional Facilities* (U.S. Department of Justice, Office of Justice Programs, June 1989). For the exceptions see p. 41 of the report. Compare the 1988 report with the *1989 Update* issued in May 1990. See also "Inescapable Problem: AIDS in Prison," *JAMA*, December 11, 1987, p. 3215.
25. Still the most arresting account of this period is Shilts' *And The Band Played On*.
26. The National Academy issued a 390-page report criticizing the President for lack of leadership. See *National Journal*, August 30, 1986, p. 2044, and November 8, 1986, p. 2733.
27. The total amount appropriated for the period commencing October 1, 1988 for the 1989 fiscal year totaled $1.5 billion.
28. "MD Relates Reasons He Left AIDS Panel," *American Medical News*, December 25, 1987, p. 2.
29. *Report of the Presidential Commission on the Human Immunodeficiency Virus*, submitted to the President of the United States, June 24, 1988.
30. Ibid., Appendix B.

31. *National Journal*, August 6, 1988, p. 2189.
32. For a summary analysis of the Presidential Commission report see *National Journal*, June 11, 1988. Also, *Congressional Quarterly*, August 6, 1988, p. 2189.
33. As an example, Representative Dannemeyer's attempts to add restrictive amendments to the House bill appropriating funds to fight AIDS were supported by 36 Republicans and 1 Democrat (Rep. Hall of Texas). The amendments were defeated 369 to 37. *Congressional Quarterly*, June 18, 1989, pp. 1695 and 1698.
34. The ambiguity of the CDC categories makes it difficult to determine the real number of what type of sexual preference is involved in each classification.
35. The Bowdler brothers, from whose name we get the term *bowdlerize*, were early Victorians who published a series of "cleansed" versions of the Bible, Shakespeare, and other great works. These editions eliminated all direct and indirect references to anything remotely resembling sex or passion so that the "fairest maiden" could read these otherwise uplifting works without embarrassment.
36. This attitude continues into the Bush administration. In October 1989 Assistant Secretary for Public Health Kay James blocked the publication of a PHS AIDS-education pamphlet on the use of condoms because it did not make clear that condoms can fail and that abstinence was the only answer. Anthony Lewis, "Bush and the Zealots," *New York Times*, October 19, 1989, p. 31.
37. See Rebecca Voelker, "Teens Seen as Next Group of New AIDS Cases," *American Medical News*, June 16, 1989, p. 11; Gina Kolata, "AIDS Is Spreading in Teen-Agers, A New Trend Alarming to Experts," *New York Times*, October 8, 1989, p. 1.
38. For summaries of the session on AIDS see the May 24, 1989 coverage in the following: *San Antonio Light, Houston Chronicle, The Austin American-Statesman, Dallas Morning News*. The Texas caseload and seroprevalence rankings are from the September 1989 *AIDS Surveillance Report* of the Federal Centers for Disease Control. The cumulative total for Texas is 7289 reported cases, 13.7 cases/100,000 population, and a per capita expenditure of 11 cents.
39. The focus of substance abuse is, of course, IV drug use. However, it should be kept in mind that both alcohol and marijuana use are definitely implicated in the spread of AIDS in that both lower or eliminate the cautions and/or inhibitions that might otherwise encourage safer sex.
40. Gary Slutkin *et al.*, "The Effect of AIDS on the TB Problem and TB Programs," in Fleming, *The Global Impact of AIDS*, Chap. 4.
41. For a summary of provisions see *Congressional Quarterly*, October 22, 1988, pp. 3068–71. The formal designation of the AIDS provisions is: Title II of the Labor and Health and Human Services of Act of 1989.
42. A trial survey was commenced in the fall of 1989 in Dallas County, Texas. The Department of Health and Human Services mailed letters to 3400 households, soliciting their participation. This first attempt was really the culmination of administrative initiatives going back to the Reagan years rather than a direct outgrowth of the statute. However, both initiatives were and are on the same track—the effort to get better data with respect to the sexual behavior of the American population as it relates to the spread of HIV. The results of the Dallas County survey produced an estimate of 0.4% seroprevalence for adults ages 18–54. The estimated number of HIV+ is 4000 (95% confidence that the population is between 2200 and 7500). This figure is lower than previous estimates based on epidemic models.
43. At current case levels the direct care allocation amounts to approximately $1000 per patient annually. Triage thinking may have been behind the decision by

Congress, in effect, to "fake" an allocation of money for support of AZT. Congress authorized, but did not appropriate, $30 million for a continuation of the Public Health Emergency Fund that subsidizes AZT purchase. In testimony before the House oversight subcommittee with jurisdiction over the Public Health Service, the Assistant Secretary of Health, Dr. James O. Mason, told the committee that, barring new money from Congress, the only place that he could get money for AZT programs was from biomedical research, prevention programs, infant mortality, cancer, or some other portion of the health budget. *Health InfoCom Network News*, August 19, 1989, p. 9.

44. The National Institutes of Health are currently offering a program under which a health care professional can have up to $20,000 annually repaid on his/her student loan if work on NIH-sponsored AIDS research is undertaken. Program director: Marc Horowitz (301-496-0357).

45. The formula for the allocation of national money to the states is as follows: each state/territory would receive for education and prevention programs the greater of:

1. A minimum of $200,000, or
2. The amount determined equally from
   a. a percentage equal to the state's population divided by the total U.S. population; and
   b. a percentage equal to the number of new AIDS cases reported by the state to the CDC, divided by the total new cases nationally.
3. In addition, states that register 1% or more of the total national AIDS cases must pass on at least one-half the national money they receive to migrant, community health, or private nonprofit ASOs.

46. The Americans with Disabilities Act extended the antidiscrimination provisions of the Civil Rights Act of 1964, the Rehabilitation Act of 1973, and the Fair Housing Act of 1988 (*Congressional Quarterly*, May 13, 1989, p. 1121). Its extension of the concept of "disability" to PWAs followed the line of reasoning suggested by U.S. Supreme Court Justice Brennan, who stated in *School Board of Nassau County, Florida v. Arline*, 480 U.S. 273 (1987), "The fact that *some* persons who have contagious diseases may pose a serious health threat to others under certain circumstances does not justify excluding from the coverage of the Act [Rehabilitation Act of 1973] all persons with actual or perceived contagious diseases." Justice Brennan explicitly excludes AIDS from his argument, stating that it was not before the court in this case, but his line of argument could be and was applied later to AIDS by the Congress in drafting the Americans with Disabilities Act.

47. The U.S. Supreme Court in *School Board of Nassau County, Florida vs. Arline*, 107 S.Ct.1123 (1987), ruled that Section 504 of the Rehabilitation Act applied to a case of tuberculosis with reasoning that clearly would apply to AIDS as well. The Department of Justice, which initially held that AIDS was not a "handicap" under the Act, changed its position in October 1988. The Americans with Disabilities Act of 1989 picks up this development and embodies it in statutory terms.

48. The ruling was an application of Sec. 504 of the *Rehabilitation Act of 1973*. "SA Nursing Homes Discriminating," *San Antonio Express-News*, October 13, 1990, p. A1.

49. Wendy E. Parmet, *Legal Rights and Communicable Disease: AIDS, The Police*

Power and Individual Liberty, p. 14. Paper delivered at the 1988 Annual Meeting of the American Political Science Association, September 1–4, 1988. The author is an Associate Professor of Law at Northeastern University Law School.

50. For a summary of the bill see *Congressional Quarterly*, August 18, 1990, pp. 2683–86; for a review see *New York Times*, August 6, 1990, p. A12.

51. *Congressional Quarterly*, August 18, 1990, p. 2683.

52. On the other hand, the formula-grant provisions of the 1988 HOPE Act provide that funds be awarded through a single formula at the state level, instead of directly to state and municipal health departments. Federal policy is thus ambiguous, not an unusual situation.

53. See "Surveillance for Epidemics — United States," *Health InfoCom Network News* 2, no. 38 (1989): p. 14. A parallel proposal from the World Health Organization suggests the establishment of global tracking stations.

54. The Federal Centers for Disease Control estimate a rate of under-reporting from 10% to 30%. However, a report from South Carolina health authorities in 1989 indicated a 40% rate of nonreporting in that state, with a much higher likelihood of nonreporting for blacks and women than whites. "Many AIDS Cases Go Unreported," *New York Times*, November 28, 1989, p. 20. It is not a problem unique to the United States. Medical experts meeting under the auspices of the World Health Organization agreed that the same problem occurs in the Muslim countries of the Middle East. They have a significant AIDS problem but refuse publicly to acknowledge it for religious and social reasons. See *New York Times*, International, February 19, 1990, p. A5.

55. For a brief review of state legislation see Larry O. Gostin, "Public Health Strategies for Confronting AIDS," *JAMA*, March 17, 1989, p. 1621.

56. The six-month interval is necessary to eliminate the so-called window of negativity during which a recently infected person would not test positive. Only Cuba has effectively imposed a total quarantine policy. However, it should be noted that apart from this extreme measure some forms of partial quarantine are not only possible but have been tried in the United States. For example, HIV+ schoolchildren have been denied admission to school, or when admitted have been physically segregated from other children. Some states have tried to isolate individuals who refused to follow court orders to refrain from sexual activity. Insurance companies have "red flagged" entire metropolitan areas that are known to house a large gay population.

57. Stephen M. Wolinsky *et al.*, "Human Immunodeficiency Virus Type I (HIV-1) Infection, a Median of 18 Months before a Diagnostic Western Blot," *Annals of Internal Medicine* 2, no. 12 (1989): 961 *et seq*. The disturbing conclusion of this study is, "There is a long and variable interval between virus acquisition and a diagnostic serum antibody response." Previous to this study, the standard wisdom was that there might be as much as a six-month lag, but the virus would usually produce a reaction within three months.

58. The United States military spent $43 million between 1986 and 1988 to test 3.2 million people. It identified 5,890 HIV+ individuals at an average cost of $7300 each. No one asserts that its procedure identified all the positives. To project this experience to the national population involves, at minimum, a multiplication by 75, and facing the fact that a civilian population would be much more difficult to test completely and reliably.

59. The following nations have instituted some AIDS-control travel and/or immi-

gration measures. In many cases, the measures seem more attuned to domestic politics than practical public health problems: Belize, Bulgaria, China, Costa Rica, Cuba, Cyprus, Ecuador, Egypt, East Germany, Bavaria (West Germany), Greece, India, Iraq, South Korea, Kuwait, Liberia, Libya, Marshall Islands, Mongolia, Pakistan, Papua New Guinea, Philippines, Qatar, Saudi Arabia, South Africa, Soviet Union, Syria, Thailand, United Arab Emirates, United States of America. Anyone considering travel to these nations should check with the consulates to obtain the current restrictions. For a summary of the requirements as of August 1989 see *New York Times*, August 13, 1989, Travel, p. 3.

60. "Hemophilia Groups May Boycott or Move," *AIDS Treatment News*, October 20, 1989. See also *Visiting the USA: A Legal Guide for Persons with HIV* (San Francisco: National Gay Rights Advocates, 540 Castro St., CA 94110).

61. There have been sporadic quasi-quarantine methods employed, like the refusal to allow attendance of infected children or physical segregation of them in the school environment, segregation of workers in the work space or prisoners in jails, and insurance "red flagging" of whole city districts known to be the living space of homosexual populations. Most of these efforts have fallen before legal challenge.

62. See the instructive debate in the *N. Engl. J. Med.*, May 11, 1989 and November 2, 1989, inspired by the publication of "The Case for Wider Testing for HIV Infection," in vol. 320, pp. 1248–54, by F. S. Rhames and D. G. Maki.

63. *Congressional Quarterly*, August 18, 1990, p. 2685.

64. For an excellent general review of the myriad concrete problems that arise see the biweekly newsletter covering legislation, regulations, and litigation, *AIDS Policy and Law* (Washington, D.C.: Buraff Publications).

65. "Steven Joseph Envisions the Future of AIDS," *The New York Native*, June 19, 1989. The text of the Commissioner's speech to the Fifth International Conference on AIDS.

66. Currently less than one-half of state Medicaid programs support prescriptions for drugs commonly used in AIDS treatment. "Medicaid's Hodgepodge on AIDS," *New York Times*, May 25, 1989, p. B18.

67. For example, all Federal employees with overseas assignments (foreign service, peace corps, etc.), the FBI and CIA, all military, an increasing number of general admissions to hospital care, patients seeking surgical intervention (especially orthopaedic), those receiving trauma or emergency care, most life and health insurance, inmates of federal and state penitentiaries, entering aliens and those applying for amnesty, health care workers, blood or organ donors, sperm bank donors, and the newborn and their mothers. The AMA advocated an even broader requirement,"those whose history or clinical status warrant this measure [involuntary testing]."

68. "Police Seeking Man Accused of Spreading AIDS," *San Antonio Express-News*, December 9, 1990, p. A1.

69. *Congressional Quarterly*, August 18, 1990, p. 2685.

7

Into the Twenty-First
Century with AIDS

The human immunodeficiency virus has been among us for at least 40 years. In its early life it was largely restricted to remote villages of sub-Saharan Africa, and was just one more killer in a land that gave birth to many. Then it reached out to the greater world. A young man in St. Louis died of "unknown causes" in 1969, having been infected years earlier. Attending physicians were so puzzled by his array of symptoms that they stored frozen samples of his tissue and blood for later analysis; that was the end of it. Now we know that he did have HIV antibodies in his blood, that he did die of opportunistic diseases associated with AIDS, and that there were other cases here and abroad. Usually the dead were not public figures, people whose death would be a matter of public comment. When a prominent person was involved, physicians attributed death to standard causes.[1] The signals sent forth by the virus were lost within, indistinguishable from, the background noise generated by a galaxy of incurable afflictions and unaccountable deaths. Finally, by the 1980s HIV confronted physicians in sophisticated metropolitan centers with enough inexplicable cases to inspire scientific curiosity and then raise alarms. The rest is history.

We have now knowingly lived with HIV for a decade, and certain things are becoming abundantly clear. First, the epidemic involves living entities in competition, and its profile changes with the dynamics of that competition. *Biologic examples* of the process emerge from the changing incidence and impact of opportunistic infections presented by HIV+ individuals. For reasons no one understands, the incidence of Kaposi's sarcoma is dropping sharply in America, while tuberculosis is shooting up. In the early days of the epidemic, KS and PCP were the two most common expressions of AIDS. Now there is a rising incidence of *mycobacterium avium* complex, toxoplasmosis, crytococcal infections, and lymphomas. People are still dying, but of different causes.[2] *Geographic examples* of the dynamic can be found in Asia. Throughout the 1980s this part of the globe seemed relatively unaffected. Epidemiologists talked of a different "pattern" of spread, and Asian politicians preened themselves on the cultural virtues that were, seemingly, holding the virus at bay. Now the virus is spreading rapidly; the "virtue" barrier turned out to be nothing more than a time lag.[3] Within the continental United States those parts of the nation previously untouched are losing their immunity. Until 1984 five U.S. cities accounted for 63% of the cases; by 1990 their share had dropped to 38%, and the virus was found to be moving into other cities as well as rural America with sufficient speed to inspire a specially funded congressional study.[4] *Demographic examples* can be drawn from the data, which indicate that the rate of new cases in the American homosexual population is decreasing, while the rate is dramatically increasing within the IV drug culture, among women, and among teens.[5] In the next 15 years it is likely that the American epidemic will come to parallel the African/Caribbean one and become a dominantly heterosexual phenomenon. The twists and turns AIDS may take in the future no one can surely know. However, it is certain that HIV, like so many other microparasites, is now irreversibly part of the global human culture. It has joined the human race, and will never just "go away."

Second, AIDS is far more than a new or recently named illness caused by a heretofore obscure and secreted virus; it is an event of global and historic proportions that touches every aspect of human existence. Our economies, our politics, our families and churches, our basic attitudes and life styles are all being profoundly influenced.

Finally, we are at the beginning, not the end, of this event. Dr. Jonathan Mann, director of the International AIDS Center at Harvard, put the situation bluntly in 1990, "The worst is yet to come."[6] At the beginning of the decade there were over 280,000 reported AIDS cases from 153 nations, 560,000 estimated AIDS cases, and a projection of 5 million to 10 million infected worldwide.[7] No one can do more than statistically estimate how many people will be infected with HIV, will progress to AIDS, and will die as we move into the early years of the twenty-first century. Different assumptions about behavior change, developing medical technologies, and the size of the existing pool of infected individuals affect everyone's forecasts. One of the more convincing studies I have seen postulates three scenarios for America by the year 2002: a "worst case" figure of 14,553,000 HIV infected, a "best case" figure of 1,583,000 (approximately the present figure), and a "middle" estimate of 5,861,000, which the authors, in an "optimistic" frame, hope will be the correct figure.[8] Another mathematical model projects a cumulative total of 7 million Americans infected over the next 20 years.[9] The Federal Centers for Disease Control anticipate an American caseload of 365,000 by the end of 1992. Health care costs will be roughly $50 billion annually in the United States alone by mid-decade. Whichever set of figures proves ultimately to be right, clearly the closing decade of the twentieth century and the opening decade of the twenty-first will be the time of AIDS. It will be a time during which the human immunodeficiency virus will come to play a part in the life of every person reading these words. Some of its effects are clearly foreseeable, others are not.

AIDS AND HEALTH CARE TECHNOLOGY

The more easily foreseeable effects are in medicine and medical care. Biomedical research has been mobilized for a forced march on AIDS. Viral research, which would normally have taken decades, is being compressed into years. It took 40 years of poliovirus research to accumulate the amount of detailed information scientists have developed in the past six years on HIV. Just a few years ago the virus was a complex, retroviral mystery and seemed virtually invulnerable to attack. Its multitude of interactions within the human system gave it so many fronts to attack us that it seemed impossible to cover them all. Now many major points of vulnerability in its life cycle are being isolated and defined by virologists. If anyone ever questioned the importance of basic research, the unravelling of HIV's secrets in our scientific laboratories should put doubts to rest; it is only with this knowledge that we will be able to devise effective counterattacks.[10]

A concrete manifestation of the improved state of knowledge can be seen in the changing perceptions on vaccines. In the 1980s scientists were uniformly pessimistic about the possibilities of an effective vaccine of any kind before the twenty-first century. By 1990 that attitude had given way to guarded optimism, as several developments suggest that not only is a treatment or therapeutic vaccine possible, but more probable than previously believed.[11] The preventive vaccine continues to remain elusive. At the beginning of the 1990s there were 11 vaccine trials under way, with funding of $24 million.[12] In addition, there are hundreds of experimental programs across the country testing the efficacy of some 70 drugs and/or combinations thereof (see Appendix 2).[13] Announcements made by Dr. Jonas Salk and others at the Sixth International Conference on AIDS, which met in San Francisco during June 1990, indicated some successes in initial vaccine trials.

The last decade of the twentieth century opened with the encouraging discovery that low-dose AZT, administered to asymptomatic PWAs, may slow the rate of progression to AIDS.[14] And what is true for AZT seems also to hold for a number of therapies. A consensus of medical opinion is developing that the most effective course is early treatment, as soon as possible following infection and before overt symptoms (indicating an entrenched infection) begin to appear. This development makes it possible, for the first time, unreservedly to advise individuals to take HIV tests. Prior to 1989 a positive test result was all pain and no gain for the individual. He or she faced the trauma of knowing, without the ability to do anything about it. Now early intervention treatments can buy precious time for millions of infected persons in the 1990s, but, obviously, only if they know they need them.[15] Dr. Mathilde Krim, formerly a researcher at the Sloan-Kettering Cancer Center and a founding co-chairperson of the American Foundation for AIDS Research (AMFAR), stated the present situation in a recent interview: "Within my lifetime, people with AIDS may live long, normal lives, receiving regular treatments."[16]

Because of AIDS research, scientists are beginning to make significant advances in our understanding and ability to cope with many other intractable and terminal viral ailments.[17] In addition, important changes are being forged in medical training, research networking, care of the terminally ill, and drug testing protocols.[18] In all these areas, but especially in drug testing, AIDS is driving the scientific community to consider techniques and possibilities that it would have rejected out of hand just a few years ago. The future care of everyone will benefit from these advances.[19]

Not least among new developments is the emergence of the "informed patient." The standard model of the doctor-patient relationship in the pre-AIDS era was one in which the patient deferentially accepted the *ex cathedra* diagnoses of his benign and all-knowing physician. All that changed with AIDS. Because of the newness of the disease, the physician had little genuine expertise; there was precious little to have. Furthermore, in America the epidemic struck first at the urban homosexual community, which has a highly educated, professional upper class. Patients drawn from such origins, and under a death sentence, were not easily put off with Latinized "medi-speak" concealing the reality that no one knew much about AIDS. A new, refreshing, and sometimes painful candor, as well as a new style of patient-doctor collaboration in fighting disease is rapidly emerging as the model for the future. As one physician put it after attending the International AIDS Conference in Montreal, "When I went to [the meeting], I was flanked on either side by a half a dozen of my own patients reading the same posters I read. I don't see an end to that. I see patients becoming more and more empowered to be involved in the process, and that's a good thing."[20]

The restructuring involves more than the private patient-doctor connection, reaching to a public or civil relationship as well. PWAs are gaining access to channels of medical information and decision-making that have always been closed to the nonprofessional. PWA groups are now part of the process by which testing protocols are developed and drugs are tested and distributed. The national government has responded to the demand for authoritative information by inaugurating a public health "first"—open-access data banks both for the professional health care worker and for the concerned citizen. Clearly, the national government has accepted a major responsibility for the level and quality of public knowledge on the epidemic. Any person wishing information about the disease or current clinical drug trials should phone 1-800-874-2572 or 1-800-243-7012 (TTD/TDY), or write the National AIDS Information Clearinghouse, P.O. Box 6003, Rockville, MD 20850.[21]

In the late 1990s these developments may eventually start to contain AIDS with a variety of medical and public health strategies. Gradually it will be reduced to the status of the most serious disease that lurks in the shadow of human sexual behavior, but not an inevitably fatal one in the short term.[22] Perhaps by then we will have learned to live with HIV, rather than die from it. Eventually all of us will look back, as did Dr. Russell V. Lee, reflecting upon his involvement as a young intern in the great flu epidemic of 1918: "We were humbled by our incapacities, but challenged by the responsibilities. [It was] . . . a great teacher, but a dear one."[23]

AIDS may be a great teacher in another sense. It is obliging us, as citizens, to consider some hard and uncomfortable questions about the connection between medical/scientific intervention, private ethics, and public policy. It shares this role with the debate over abortion and the use of extraordinary life maintenance equipment. As we move into the twenty-first century, medical tests and genetic engineering will become available, making it possible to control eugenically for hereditary disease, as well as for other less clearly disadvantageous traits (like left-handedness, for example). We will need to consider how far we care, or dare, to go in playing God with the evolution of our species. Clearly, we will have the technological skill.

We will need convincing answers to questions as to whether we should make use of the entire array of applicable medical interventions, regardless of cost, for people who present terminal, incurable illnesses. Should we discriminate in the allocation of services based on the patient's age, gender, wealth, occupation, mode of getting the disease, or previous or possible future social contribution? Should we treat the business person but not the street person, the infant but not the adult, the heterosexual but not the homosexual? As taxpayers should we pay the bill for the education of a child born with a disease that makes it unlikely that he/she will live to the age of 20? Should such a birth be aborted, or, if not, who pays for the extraordinary costs of life maintenance, the public or the parents? Given the short supply of transplant organs, should alcoholics get new livers or heavy smokers new hearts? These difficult questions are the raw material of personal, medical, and social debates; AIDS is helping to propel them into the public forum where, ultimately, they must be resolved by the people whose lives will be enhanced or diminished by the answers.

Furthermore, AIDS will require us to search our hearts to decide how much we are willing to pay for some of our ancient beliefs; in effect, it is asking us to calculate the human mortality costs of preserving traditional dogmas. From time immemorial political and ecclesiastical officials have been willing to sacrifice live people to protect the purity of abstract doctrine, ignoring the fact that there is no necessary relationship between logic and real life. Perhaps the devastation of AIDS, when its full impact is felt, will help convince us that it is time to stop all forms of human sacrifice, the subtle as well as the blatant. We do need logic to form a scaffolding for thought, but it ought never be confused with the substance of it. Life or death, nature's binary, are the only absolute values; all else is negotiable.

A clear example bedeviling Catholics arises from their opposition to the use of condoms. The church's need to maintain the ban on condoms (to preserve doctrinal purity) runs squarely into the reality that, at this time, condoms are the only reasonably effective protection against transmission of any pathogen that can be sexually transmitted, including HIV. Clearly they are not perfect, and can even have tragic results in case of failure, but they are the best that we have. That they do not work perfectly is no argument against them; nothing does, save a perfect, abstinent chastity that not even the priesthood achieves. Nor is the argument convincing that we must mount a vigorous educational campaign on the virtues of abstinence; all history testifies, and every teacher knows, that there are limits to the ability of education to effect basic behavioral change, particularly in the short run. The blunt truth is that the cost of maintaining doctrinal purity will be reckoned in lives lost.

Furthermore, the epidemic will put our health care delivery nonsystem under such an increasingly heavy strain that eventually we will be compelled to rationalize it, nationalize it, and guarantee Americans access to care.[24] Already the American Medical Association and the American College of Physicians are calling for a reexamination and overhaul of our health care delivery system.[25] Canada, Australia, and other nations have provided necessary drugs like AZT from the beginning, accepting a responsibility about which we still vacillate. AIDS will force hard decisions upon us. For example, it will compel us to decide whether we wish to continue spending 40% of all Medicare funds on patients with no hope of recovery during the last six months of their lives, or whether it is socially just to continue spending 55% of the nation's health care dollars on 5% of the population.

Can we continue to leave 50 million Americans with no effective health coverage?[26]

AIDS may well be one of the stimuli that will prod our reluctant nation to provide an effective level of health care as a statutory entitlement, and it may be the force that will demote the profit motive from its present commanding position as the system's driver. Expanding the reach of health insurance will not be as radical a change as many Americans think because we are almost there now. The national government already makes beneficial coverage available for all members of the military, all veterans, all members of Congress and their staffs, the President and Vice President and their staffs, the executive and independent regulatory bureaucracies, the court system and its supporting staff, the elderly, and the disabled or handicapped. In addition, most political and administrative state employees, employees of larger businesses, and teachers at all levels in public and private systems are covered by some form of insurance. Essentially, national health insurance means extending benefits already enjoyed by the bulk of the work force to everyone.

The biggest problem will not be extension, but cost containment, since that is tied to the profit motive. All existing actors in the system, physicians, hospitals, and drug companies, stand to gain from keeping things as they are; there are no incentives for anyone in health care to control and contain costs. Consequently, unless we are willing to pay a major share of our tax dollars to the health care industry, the currently dominant influence of the profit motive will have to be severely diminished by statutory regulation of medical service and drug pricing.

AIDS and Cultural Values

More problematic, more difficult to discern are the social impacts. One that may emerge is an America where the homosexual no longer need hide—the elimination of the last great outcast group. Truly this would be a radical change, since homosexuals have had to conceal their sexual identity since the intolerant, sex-negative Judeo-Christian culture displaced the tolerant Greco-Roman one.

Every nation has its outcasts, people who suffer severe legal and social discrimination because of their gender, race, religion, ethnicity, or class. It is one of the more destructive tendencies of our species to classify people into "them" and "us," "Greek" and "Barbarian" categories. Mainstream Americans built social and legal discriminations around many groups—Irish, Mormons, Catholics, Orientals, Slavs, Turks and Middle Easterners, Central and Eastern Europeans, American Indians, and Mexican Americans.[27] Jews, blacks, women, and homosexuals were the largest groups subject to pervasive discrimination. In each case, the white Anglo-Saxon male majority rationalized its action on egregious Biblical interpretations. Jews were responsible for the execution of Christ, blacks bore the mark of Cain, women were derivative of and intended to be servants of men, and homosexuals acted contrary to the "order of nature." Jews, blacks, and women have been beating down the barriers by using every technique from outright physical assault to the choreographed violence of litigation. They made little real progress until they mobilized in their interests.

In the next decade, a major social significance of AIDS may be the mobilization of America's millions of homosexuals and the creation of the sense of community that is the base for effective politics. AIDS has made political action, and its consequent visibility, a condition of survival. It has dragged many gays out of their protective closets and diminished the significance of the straight world's homophobic sanctions. Before the AIDS epidemic there was little more than the loose network of the Metropolitan Community Churches that could be called a gay community infrastructure. Today an elaborate collection of political action groups, businesses, social clubs, community service and health care organizations, churches, and publications have emerged to respond to an increasingly visible and vocal gay population.[28]

In this epidemic, gays have become an important influence in compelling a conservative government and biomedical establishment to reevaluate its traditional approaches and techniques of drug evaluation and delivery. For example, one of the most important documents delivered at Montreal's Fifth International Conference on AIDS was "A National AIDS Treatment and Research Agenda," prepared by the AIDS Coalition to Unleash Power (ACT UP). This study inspired a major reevaluation of procedures by the National Institutes of Health. Only a few years ago it would have been inconceivable that government agencies (especially large bureaucracies like the National Institutes of Health and the Federal Drug Administration) would respond directly to an openly gay pressure group, especially one that had stormed New York's St. Patrick's Cathedral to protest Cardinal O'Connor's orthodox homophobia.[29] ACT UP is an activist, confrontational gay pressure group focusing on AIDS issues. It has adapted Carry Nation's advice to the American farmer, "Raise less corn, and more hell."[30] If it can formulate broader, longer-term goals, it could be the foundation for a gay version of the Jewish Anti-Defamation League.

In the 1990s gays, prodded by AIDS, will likely be more insistent and more organizationally effective in their petition for reconsideration by the culture. They will demand status acceptance, if not approval, with all that such acceptance implies in terms of benefits and protection under the Constitution and laws of the United States. In politics, mainstream churches, and the military, the one-time absolute barrier stemming from being a known homosexual is under siege and giving way.[31] In the twenty-first century it is likely that America's secular and religious intelligentsia will finally and utterly abandon the defense of our ancient, destructive mythologies. We then will be able to welcome in our last major outcast group.[32] Supreme Court Justice Harlan's famous 1896 dissenting comment will finally become the law of the land: "The Constitution . . . neither knows nor tolerates classes among its citizens."[33]

Yet, it is not beyond the realm of possibility that, as the epidemic spreads, Americans led by home-grown demagogues, of whom we have always had a plentiful supply, could violently react against the groups they identify as the source of the epidemic. By 2005, projecting from the current HIV+ pool, the epidemic will have a very different focus than it had in the early years. The current ratio of heterosexual to homosexual afflicted (about 33% heterosexual, 63% homosexual, the remainder pediatric) will reverse. In addition there will be a much larger component of females. If current projections are correct, it will probably become an epidemic of the "marginal classes" (blacks, Hispanics, gays, and ghetto teens), as far as white, middle-class America is concerned. The potential in this situation for the surfacing and exacerbation of class, racial, and religious hatreds is obvious. The scapegoating that led to the herding and burning of Jews during the Black Death could recur. It would require a level of panic sufficient to threaten our basic institutions, but it could happen. It is painful but wise to remember that Adolph Hitler and his Nazis were not a perversion of the Western cultural tradition. On the contrary, they were the apocalyptic administrators of some of its most consistent hatreds.

The Nazi extermination of homosexuals and Jews was the tragic apotheosis of the Old Testament, Greek, and early Christian doctrine, which taught that people should be separated into "chosen" or "natural" categories of moral superiority and inferiority, and that those who were inferior could be dispensed with. Our surest protection against such a movement in America will be the selection of national leaders capable of exerting a strong but compassionate leadership, the kind we associate with Lincoln.

AIDS is raising questions at this most basic and profound level. It is not a judgment of God, but it most definitely is a trial. It will be a great test to determine whether the ruling white, heterosexual community can move beyond the myopia of self, which so easily flows from power, and throw off the prejudices that have been cancerous within our culture for over 2000 years.[34] As Karl Mannheim pointed out in *Ideology and Utopia*, when people are immersed in a certain ideology or religion they lose their ability to see certain facts; they are blinded not by optic degeneration, but by internalized templates that allow only parts of the real world to pass, just as polarized lenses filter some of the light.[35] It is not easy to shatter these lenses once installed; it is not easy to alter the mindset of an entire culture, no matter how wrongheaded the ideas may be. But it can be done. Between 1300 and 1800 Western church-state officials (mostly male) burned alive hundreds of thousands of witches (mostly female); now most of us no longer even believe in witches. AIDS sets the stage for one of the great challenges of the twenty-first century, one that will require all our goodwill and intellectual resources—the challenge of exorcising homophobia from the mind of America.

AIDS AND THE SOCIAL CONTRACT

Many factors contribute to the changes of history, frequently in unexpected and unforeseeable ways. For example, epidemics crippled the French military presence in the Caribbean, so Napoleon wisely sold Jefferson the Louisiana Territory he could no longer defend. America, until then an insignificant shoestring republic tied to the east coast of a vast continent, was launched upon one of history's most extensive and successful territorial conquests. It was like winning an unbelievably rich lottery at the beginning of one's career. Similarly, the great fourteenth and fifteenth century visitations of the bubonic plague helped kill feudalism, especially in England. So many people died, especially in the urban areas, that a manpower shortage developed which, in turn, raised the value of urban labor. In spite of legal measures designed to "keep them down on the farm," the serf left the feudal estates to seek a better life in the city. Looking from our time forward, AIDS might well accelerate very basic changes that are taking place in the organization of the global community.

We are told that the Great Wall of China is the only human artifact observable from space. It is appropriate that this be so. The construction of walls dividing people from people has been one of the most enduring traits of the human species. We have built them of everything, from the concrete blocks of the Berlin Wall, through electronic walls in space, to elaborate codes of prejudice like America's Jim Crow and South Africa's apartheid laws. The walls are even present within the community of those dying from AIDS; they can be encountered within any AIDS Service Organization trying to meet the interests of all kinds of clients. There is a gulf, unbridgeable even by common affliction and destiny, between various groups of PWAs—for example, those from the gay middle and upper classes, and those from poor circumstances or from the streets. There is little understanding or sympathy between the IV and non-IV groups. And those who acquired the virus through blood transfusion tend to keep strictly to themselves, mounting separate "innocent victim" campaigns for assistance from the government. I suppose that, from Troy to the present, the building of garrison, city, national, class, religious, and ethnic walls has had some survival value for the world's cultures. All of our great moral leaders from Christ to Schopenhauer, Gandhi, and Martin Luther King tried to teach us otherwise, but we nonetheless built walls, walls, and more walls.

Tampering with our walls is a traumatic and dangerous business, for we have entire cultures invested in them. Still, the fact remains that they no longer serve to protect us from anything more than the necessary next phase of cultural evolution, the development of a global human community neither confined nor deformed by national or psychological boundaries. Everywhere there are signs that old walls are tumbling down. The disintegration of both the American and Soviet empires opens rich new possibilities of East-West exchange. The gradual realization of the European Economic Community, and the proposal of many others, will intertwine our various interests such that violent conflict will be suicidal.

Signs of the coming times are the emergence of the World Trade Centers network to promote direct international contact between small businesses, and, of course, the gradual domination of all economies by the new leviathans, multinational corporations and banks. Profound structural changes at the top, like the cartelization of global commerce, are matched in importance at the "people" level by population movement in a volume unprecedented in history. On every continent millions of migrant laborers wash across boundaries like tidal waves. Today's workers flee poverty in their homelands, just as England's serfs fled the feudal estates six centuries ago. North America's experience with migration from Mexico and Central America shows that quotas and boundary checks are no more effective a dam to the flow than were the statutes of Edward III in 1351.[36] Besides, the immigrants are wanted! Flying over their heads are the very businesspeople who will hire them.

[The increasing interconnectedness of economies and peoples means that we can no longer fence out problems.]The weakness of Latin American economies and the global decline of petroleum values spread so much sickness in American lending institutions that now only the entire taxpaying public can generate enough revenue to defray the recovery costs. Likewise, America cannot contain its share of a global AIDS epidemic without attending to patients abroad. In 1987 Prof. Thomas H. Weller, Nobel laureate, in an article that should be read by everyone concerned with AIDS, predicted that the epidemic will not be contained until we accept two facts: (1) that AIDS threatens and affects everyone on the planet, not just politically impotent minorities like New York junkies, Bangkok prostitutes, or Mexico City's homeless street urchins,[37] and (2) that it cannot be conceptualized as just a public health problem to be dealt with by health measures alone.[38] He points out that while AIDS is, on its surface, a problem of public health, it is actually far more. Weller contends that a successful strategy of containment must attack a broad front of late twentieth century dilemmas, problems that are reflections of the gross maldistribution of wealth both within and among nations.

For example, AIDS has killed Haitians and Haiti's critical tourist industry; it threatens to do the same in Thailand. It will probably lead to major ecological collapse in central Africa as villages lose the manpower to keep land under cultivation. AIDS will probably undermine all the advancements made in Third World economies since the 1950s and nullify the effect of billions in foreign aid over the last 25 years. Instead of a brighter, more viable economic future, the view from AIDS is famine. No Third World nation can afford the multimillion-dollar cost of a thoroughly screened blood supply; without help they will necessarily remain a continuing source of HIV infection. Typical treatment for AIDS in Tanzania, which has one physician per 32,000 people, is bed rest and a few aspirin. The total budget of Zaire's largest hospital is comparable to the cost of treating 10 patients in America. The United States spent $43 million to identify 5890 infected military, a sum greater than central Africa's total health budget.[39]

These kinds of discrepancies are commonplace between rich and poor nations, but with AIDS it is no longer just a matter of the number of phones, indoor toilets, or even caloric intake per capita. Clearly it is now a case where the "haves" must help the "have nots" if they are concerned with the state of their own health. Self-interest dictates that the great nations launch an integrated global strategy, or AIDS will return again and again, as did the bubonic plague, to infect them.[40] Modern China, using the controls of a police state, tried to build a wall of protection against the spread of AIDS just as, long ago, it tried to shut out the Mongol armies. Both attempts failed.[41] We cannot fence out the world's politico-economic woes, nor its diseases. Both are endemic to the body of Mother Earth.[42]

Nor can AIDS be fenced in! Every nation has what the politicians like to call "pockets of poverty," suggesting by the imagery of the phrase that almost everyone is fat and happy. Nationally and globally, it is a lie. What we really have are "pockets of wealth" sewed with threads of pain and deprivation on an otherwise poor fabric. Politically and economically, America is owned and operated by a very small percentage of its population, and America has an equitable distribution of wealth and power compared with nations like Mexico or Saudi Arabia.[43]

So what? What is the connection to an epidemic? The connection is that the conditions and services that make for a healthy population, as well as the literacy and education that make that population susceptible to health warnings, are closely tied to significant private discretionary resources. The middle and lower classes, the majority of all nations, have few, if any.

Without a broad-based attack on the epidemic, the American and global underclass will bear a disproportionate share of the epidemic's burden in a manifestly unjust way, and class injustice has a way of coming back to haunt the societies that perpetrate it—as every white American ought to know. It is an exercise in self-deception and futility to frame policy that addresses AIDS without also targeting poverty, illiteracy, drug addiction, and, ultimately, the barren, empty lives that result. Those fortunate enough to live in the upper Manhattans of this world cannot wall in the huge areas of hopelessness. The urban ghettoes will function as encapsulated foci of endemicity; they will be the reservoirs from which AIDS will draw ever renewed vitality.

The problems resulting from growing interconnectedness will be more acute in just a few years. It is possible that by the year 2000, 75% of the world's 5 billion people will live in urban areas; in 1900 it was over 75% rural. As noted in Chapter 3, epidemics are metropolitan events. Cities are and always have been the playgrounds of epidemics. If we continue to develop sprawling and pestilential *barrios, favellas,* ghettoes, and slums like Calcutta's ironically named City of Joy,[44] we will guarantee the continued vitality of not only the human immunodeficiency virus but other, perhaps deadlier, agents now waiting in the wings. One answer to the problems that arise in living next-door to poverty—one that will be tried—will be to create physical and electronic barriers, a new form of *cordon sanitaire*, around the comfortable classes. Walled islands of wealth will be scattered in the troubled ocean of poverty. We try, rather ineffectively, to use these now to frustrate the car thief and house burglar—but how does one fence a virus in or out?

The AIDS epidemic in the next two or three decades should provide us with the stimulus to depreciate the things that divide us, and search for ways as a global family to stop the destroyer within our collective body. Today Americans read about 160,000 American cases; all too soon the figure will be 1 million, and there will be millions more abroad. Our leaders must work the subtle alchemy needed to transmute our interconnectedness into a global community. Perhaps only the threat posed by the human immunodeficiency virus, with its weighty sanction of mass death, can provide the incentive to abandon our walls, to set aside our ancient investment in hatred, prejudice, and separateness. We can then jointly attack our common non-national, non-religious, non-racial, non-human adversary. We can realize our most noble aspirations and build a new global and humane union. Changes of this magnitude in human organization are so basic and profound that they find an analog only in the movement of the very earth we walk upon, the shift of major continental plates. Whether this be our path or not, whether we succeed or not, we will at least come to understand the truth of Bishop Cyprian's final thought on the epidemic of his time, and its application to ours: "[H]ow suitable, how necessary it is that this plague and pestilence which seems horrible and deadly, searches out the justice of each and every one, and examines the minds of the human race."

Notes

1. Very technically speaking, there were no "AIDS" or "HIV" deaths prior to 1987. Before that, deaths were routinely described by such recognized medical categories as "cell-mediated immunity deficiencies" or "*Pneumocystis carinii*." The international standard for ascribing the cause of death is the World Health Organization's *Manual of the International Statistical Certification of Diseases, Injuries, and Causes of Death* (Geneva, 1977). The manual was updated to include HIV infection in 1987. See: Federal Centers for Disease Control, *Mortality and Morbidity Weekly Report* (MMWR), human immunodeficiency virus (HIV) infection codes: official authorized addendum ICD-9-CM, 1987:36 (no. S-7). This classification time lag was the basis for some conflicts of ascription among private attending physicians, public coroners, and the media in "celebrity" deaths. For the 1987 revision of the syndrome, see MMWR, 1987:36 (no. 1S).
2. See the report of Dr. Marcus Conant on the Sixth International Conference on AIDS, San Francisco, June 1990, in *AIDS Treatment News*, July 6, 1990.
3. Lecture of Dr. Anthony Fauci, Director of NIAID, December 6, 1989, National Institutes of Health Clinical Center, as summarized in *Washington HIV News*, January 1990.
4. *The 57th Annual Meeting of the United States Conference of Mayors, Task Force on AIDS, 1989 Report.* And see "AIDS Enters Rural Areas; 150 [Texas] Counties Report Cases, *San Antonio Express-News*, May 7, 1990, p. 7c. The rate of increase in new cases in rural America is 37%, while the urban rate is 5%. Congress funded a special study in Title IV of the Ryan White AIDS Act of 1990.
5. See Ronald Smothers, "Spread of AIDS in Rural Areas Testing Georgia," *New York Times*, April 18, 1990, p. A8. See also U.S. Department of Health and Human Services, *HIV/AIDS Surveillance: U.S. AIDS Cases Reported Through January 1990* (Washington, D.C.: February 1990). The World Health Organization predicts that by 2000 A.D. three-fourths of HIV infections, or 80% of the worldwide total, will be from heterosexual contact. *HIC Medical News*, December 9, 1990.
6. Dr. Mann's address to an international AIDS symposium in Atlanta, GA, in September 1990 (Associated Press). *San Antonio Express-News*, September 28, 1990, p. A13.
7. *AIDS Surveillance Report* (update), July 1, 1990, World Health Organization. And see Dr. James Chin, Chief, Surveillance, Forecasting and Impact Assessment, WHO Global Programme on AIDS, "Understanding the Figures," *World Health: The Magazine of the World Health Organization*, October 1989. In the same issue: Dr. Jonathan Mann, "Global AIDS in the 1990s."
8. William B. Johnston and Kevin R. Hopkins, *The Catastrophe Ahead* (New York: Praeger, 1990), p. 7, Table 1.1. The authors also break the total projections down into white, black, and Hispanic subgroups.

9. Rebecca Voelker, "Model Predicts Huge Jump in AIDS in Coming Years," *American Medical News*, December 22/29, 1989, p. 4. Mathematician Yakov Fuxman developed his models in response to insurance industry needs for long-term projections. The methods used by the Federal Centers for Disease Control cannot accurately forecast for the long term. The Centers projection anticipates 365,000 cases by the end of 1992.

10. See Broder, "The Life-Cycle of the Human Immunodeficiency Virus as a Guide to New Therapies," in Vincent de Vita *et al.* (eds.), *AIDS: Etiology, Diagnosis, Treatment and Prevention*, pp. 79–87. Gina Kolata, "AIDS Research Finds 13 Vulnerable Spots in Virus Life Cycle," *New York Times*, October 2, 1990, p. B6, summarizes Dr. Broder's most recent article on the same subject which appeared in *Science*, October 1990.

11. "Hope for AIDS Vaccines," *Science*, October 6, 1989, p. 23.

12. See lecture of Dr. Anthony Fauci, NIAID, December 6, 1989, at NIH Clinical Center, Washington, D.C., as summarized in *Washington HIV News* 1, no. 4 (January 1990). Also see John Capri, "The AIDS Vaccine Front Expanding," *Medical Tribune*, March 8, 1990.

13. For summaries of experimental protocols and drug investigations in operation in the first half of 1990 see *Washington HIV News*, August 1989 and February 1990; and *Health Info-com Network Newsletter*, May 16, 1990.

14. The original research upon which the new low-dose protocols are based is Paul Volberding *et al.*, "Zidovudine in Asymptomatic Human Immunodeficiency Infection," *N. Engl. J. Med.*, April 5, 1990, p. 941. And see "Early Treatment for HIV: The Time Has Come!" (editorial), same issue; and Gay Men's Health Crisis, "AZT Update: News from San Francisco," *Treatment Issues*, August 30, 1990. However, it should be noted that early, low-dose protocols may not affect the AIDS death rate. See "Federal Study Questions Ability of the Drug AZT to Delay AIDS," *New York Times*, February 15, 1991, p. A1.

15. Remarks of Dr. Basil Vereldzis, *Washington HIV News*, January 1990. And see "Long Term AZT Treatment," *Internal Medicine, World Report*, December 1, 1989, p. 22; and "Low-Dose AZT plus Acyclovir Safe for Asymptomatic HIV Infected Patients," February 1, 1990, p. 1; and "The 1989 AIDS Survey" (of primary care physicians), same issue. See also the coverage in the AMA's *American Medical News*, February 9, 1990.

16. Interview with Stephen Brewer, *New Choices*, July 1989, pp. 40–41.

17. See, for example, "The Cutting Edge: Advances in Medical Technology, Polymerase Chain Reaction Diagnostics," *Internal Medicine World Report* 5, no. 4, (1990): p. 9.

18. See William A. Check, " Growing Up Fast : A New Generation of AIDS Physicians," *Observer* (American College of Physicians), 9, no. 10 (November 1989): 1. For more expedited drug delivery resulting from the PCP/steroid treatment delay, see *New York Times*, November 14, 1990, p. A1.

19. *N. Engl. J. Med.*, November 9, 1989, pp. 1334–36. Check, "Growing up Fast." *New York Times*, "Benefits of Treating AIDS at Home," November 11, 1989, p. 26. Gina Kolata, "Radically Wider Testing of AIDS Drugs Is Urged," *New York Times*, March 26, 1990, p. A1; "Many Recommend Disputed AIDS Drug," *New York Times*, March 19, 1990, p. A13; "New System for Staging Clinical AIDS Proposed," *Internal Medicine News*, February 1–14, 1990, p. 28a. John S. James, "Toward Faster Antiviral Development: 'Rapid Screening' Trials Proposed," *AIDS Treatment News*, September 7, 1990.

20. The comments of Dr. Marcus Conant in *Internal Medicine News*, January 15–31, 1990, p. 28a.

21. This service is a U.S. Public Health Service project provided collaboratively by the Centers for Disease Control, the Food and Drug Administration, the National Institute of Allergy and Infectious Diseases of the NIH, and the National Library of Medicine. It is operated by the National AIDS Information Clearinghouse and was authorized and funded by the Omnibus 1988 Act discussed in Chapter 6.

22. One of the most interesting and potentially valuable developments is the establishment of specialized AIDS research laboratories capable of focusing world-class research efforts on the virus's vulnerable processes. An example is the AIDS Research Center of New York City, funded by private donation and government grant. See "Big Lab for AIDS to Open in Manhattan," *New York Times*, January 31, 1990, p. A20.

23. Dr. Lee's remembrance of the 1917 epidemic and his comparison to the present one are worth reading. *Internal Medicine News*, January 1–14, 1988, p. 17.

24. See the excellent summary of national health care problems and possible government interventions. "Health under the Knife," *National Journal*, March 24, 1990.

25. See "National Health Insurance, Has Its Time Come?" *Observer* (American College of Physicians) 10, no. 1 (January 1990): 1; American Medical Association, "AMA's 'Health Access America,'" *American Medical News*, March 16, 1990, p. 1.

26. Linda Marsa, "Phoenix Rising," *OMNI*, December 1989, p. 50.

27. For example, prior to the 1940s when the U.S. Supreme Court declared them unenforceable at law, most homes in the "better" areas had racially restrictive covenants upon them which effectively excluded almost everyone who was not of English/Scottish or Western European origin.

28. See the excellent summary article, Carol Matlack, "Gay Clout," *National Journal*, January 6, 1990.

29. *New York Times*, December 11, 1989, p. A17, and December 12, p. A24.

30. ACT UP was founded by the playwright Larry Kramer, among others. Kramer, who is personally fighting AIDS, was also one of the founders of the New York City's Gay Men's Health Crisis, the nation's largest single private, volunteer AIDS service organization. See his *Reports from the Holocaust: The Making of an AIDS Activist* (New York: St. Martin's Press, 1989). For a description of some ACT UP initiatives see Gina Kolata, "Advocates' Tactics on AIDS Issues Provoking Warnings of a Backlash," *New York Times*, Week In Review, March 11, 1990, p. 5E.

31. See *Newsweek*, September 25, 1989, for feature articles on homosexuality and politics. Mireya Navarro, "A Gay Man Is Ordained as an Episcopal Priest," *New York Times*, December 17, 1989, p. 24. See also *New York Times*, January 29, 1990. The unusual feature is not that a homosexual was ordained, but that an open and admitted homosexual was ordained. The priest in question is the Reverend J. Robert Williams, Episcopal diocese of Newark, NJ. Elaine Sciolino, "Report Urging that Military End Ban on Homosexuals Is Rejected," *New York Times*, October 22, 1989, p. 1.

32. The temporary suspension of editorial commentator Andy Rooney by CBS for remarks offensive to homosexuals and blacks is an example of withdrawal of powerful institutional support for inaccurate and offensive public statements

(Mr. Rooney, in effect, equated homosexual sex with unsafe sex in the context of the AIDS epidemic). In the same vein, Congress enacted and President Bush signed, in April 1990, legislation to gather data on "hate" crimes, those inspired by bigotry of any kind. Presumably this will be preparatory to legislation dealing directly with this phenomenon.

33. *Plessy v. Ferguson* (1896). Justice Harlan's original comment, like the case, related to blacks and racial segregation. The underlying premise applies to all.

34. There are hopeful signs, such as congressional consideration of bills punishing "hate crimes." See "Senate, 92–4, Wants U.S. Data on Hate Crimes Spawned by Bias," *New York Times*, February 9, 1990. Universities, including mine, are gradually recognizing gay student clubs (sometimes under court order). There are a scattering of antidiscrimination housing and benefit ordinances.

35. See Chapter 1.

36. Statute of Labourers, 25 Edward III, st.1, 1351. For a brief discussion of the impact of the Black Death on English law of the period see Thomas Pitt Taswell-Langmead, *English Constitutional History*, 10th ed. (London: Houghton, Mifflin Co., 1946), pp. 203–5.

37. A lengthy Associated Press story appearing in the *San Antonio Express-News* on November 5, 1989, talks of as many as 2 million abandoned or runaway youths in Mexico City showing signs of harboring an AIDS infection. "AIDS Stalking the Street: Lost Children of Mexico," *San Antonio Express-News*, November 5, 1989, p. 2b.

38. Thomas A. Weller, Richard Pearson Strong Professor of Tropical Public Health Emeritus, Harvard School of Public Health, "Lessons for the Control of AIDS," *Hospital Practice*, November 15, 1987, p. 41. Dr. Weller was a co-recipient of the Nobel Prize in Physiology and Medicine in 1954.

39. See the fine series of four articles by Eric Ekholm with Jon Tierney, "AIDS in Africa," which commenced in the *New York Times*, September 16, 1990, p. A1.

40. There are now about 160 private agencies in addition to the usual public health government bodies dealing with various aspects of AIDS in the developing countries. There is the beginning of some action and coordination through the Global Programme on AIDS of the World Health Organization, the Pan American Health Organization, the U.S. Agency of International Development, and the Fogarty International Center of the U.S. National Institutes of Health. So far it is only an underfunded beginning. See World Health Organization, Global Programme on AIDS, *Inventory of Nongovernmental Organizations Working on AIDS in Developing Countries* (preliminary version, 1989).

41. Sheryl WuDunn, "Outbreak of AIDS Among Drug Users Alarms China," *New York Times*, March 30, 1990, National, p. A12.

42. Recognizing this fact of international life, the U.S. Centers for Disease Control recommended in February 1990 that the United States drop AIDS from its list of illnesses that are used to bar people from visiting or immigrating. See *New York Times*, February 28, 1990, p. A15.

43. See the following analyses: James W. Lamare, *What Rules America?* (St. Paul, MN: West Publications, 1988); Michael Parenti, *Democracy for the Few*, 5th ed. (St. Martin's Press, 1989).

44. Dominique Lapierre, *The City of Joy* (New York: Warner Books, 1985).

Appendix 1

AIDS Information Resources and Further Reading

American Information Resources

AIDS Targeted Information Newletter (ATIN), published by Williams & Wilkins, P.O. Box 23291, Baltimore, MD 21203 (1-800-638-6423). A monthly annotated bibliography drawn from over 100 professional journals. This is an indispensable research tool designed for the professional researcher.

AIDS Treatment News, published by John S. James, P.O. Box 411256, San Francisco, CA 94141 (1-415-255-0588). A biweekly newsletter covering standard and alternative experimental treatments. Also concerned with public policy issues involved in clinical trials. Available by subscription.

AIDS Treatment Registry (1-212-268-4196). Current information on clinical trials in New York and New Jersey.

American Foundation for AIDS Research (AMFAR), 1515 Broadway, Suite 3601, New York, NY 10036 (1-212-719-0033). One of the major private research and resource agencies. Publishes *AIDS/HIV Treatment Directory*, a guide to approved and experimental treatments.

Body Positive, 208 West 13th St., New York, NY 10011 (1-212-633-1782). An organization of HIV + people who publish a monthly newsletter, *The Body Positive*.

Gay Men's Health Crisis, Inc., 129 West 20th St., New York, NY 10011. The nation's first and largest AIDS Service Organization publishes a number of newsletters and bulletins, most importantly *Treatment Issues*. Write to the Department of Medical Information.

Healing AIDS, 3835 20th St., San Francisco, CA 94114 (1-415-821-7646). *Healing AIDS* is a monthly magazine focusing on alternative approaches, nutritional, herbal, and so forth. Available by inexpensive subscription.

Mothers of AIDS Patients, P.O. Box 3132, San Diego, CA 92103 (619-293-3985).

National AIDS Information Clearinghouse, P.O. Box 6003, Rockville, MD 20850 (1-800-458-5231).

National Institute of Health Hotline (1-800-TRIALS-A). The hotline (AIDS Clinical Trials Information Service) for information on federally sponsored clinical trials operates Monday through Friday, 9:00 a.m. to 7:00 p.m. EST.

National Library of Medicine, *Monthly Bibliography for AIDS*. This comprehensive publication can be found in any library with a government documents section. Ask the reference librarian.

Pharmaceutical Manufacturers Association, 1100 15th St., NW, Washington, D.C. For current information on AIDS medicines, drugs, and vaccines in various stages of development and testing write: The Editor, AIDS Medicines in Development, at the above address.

Project Inform. This organization publishes a number of relevant bulletins and newsletters, such as *PI Perspective*. Call 1-800-822-7422 for information.

PWA Coalition, Inc., 31 West 26th St., New York, NY 10010 (1-212-532-0290). The PWA Coalition publishes a monthly newsletter called *PWA Coalition Newsline* written "by and for People with AIDS."

U.S. Centers for Disease Control, Aids Program, Center for Infectious Diseases, Division of HIV/AIDS, 1600 Clifton Rd., Bldg. 6, Room 285, Atlanta, GA 30333. The Centers are the source of all official statistics on AIDS. They publish the monthly *HIV/AIDS Surveillance* as well as *CDC HIV/AIDS Prevention Newsletter*, a quarterly funded under the HOPE Act which saw its first edition, vol. 1, no. 1, in October 1990. For copies write to the editors, Linda Cayton and Carol O'Connell, 1600 Clifton Road, MS/E41, Atlanta, GA 30333.

Canadian Information Resources

AIDS Calgary Awareness Association, 1021 10th Ave. SW, Suite 300, Calgary, Alberta T2R OB7, Canada (403-228-0155).

Canadian AIDS Society, 170 Laurier Ave. West, Suite 1101, Ottawa, KIP 5V5, Canada (613-230-3580).

Emergency Drug Release Program, Ottawa (613-993-3105).

Federal Center for AIDS, 301 Elgin St., 2nd Floor, Ottawa, Ontario K1A OL2, Canada.

Laboratory Center for Disease Control, Tunney's Pasture, Ottawa K1A OL2, Canada (613-998-8784).

International

World Health Organization, Surveillance, Forecasting and Impact Assessment Unit (SFI), Global Programme on AIDS, 1211 Geneva 27, Switzerland, WHO publishes a monthly, *World Health*, which covers AIDS as well as public health matters. The October 1989 issue was entirely on AIDS.

Recommended Further Reading

Johnston, William B., and Kevin R. Hopkins. *The Catastrophe Ahead, AIDS and the Case for a New Public Policy*. Published in cooperation with the Hudson Institute. New York: Praeger, 1990.

McNeill, William H. *Plagues and Peoples*. New York: Anchor Press, Doubleday, 1976.

Science, "The AIDS Issue," 239, no. 4840 (February 4, 1988).

Scientific American, 259, no. 4, October 1988, "What Science Knows about AIDS," 263, no. 2, p. 50, August 1990; "AIDS-Related Infections," John Mills and Henry Masur.

Shilts, Randy, *And the Band Played On: Politics, People, and the AIDS Epidemic.* New York: St. Martin's Press, 1987.

Other Sources

Altman, Dennis. *AIDS in the Mind of America.* New York: Doubleday, 1986.

Bateson, Mary Catherine, and Richard Goldsby. *Thinking AIDS: The Social Response to the Biological Threat.* Reading, MA: Addison-Wesley, 1988.

Blanchet, Kevin D. (ed.). *AIDS, A Health Care Management Response.* Rockville, MD: Aspen Press, 1988.

Dreuilhe, Emmanuel. *Mortal Embrace: Living with AIDS* (Linda Coverdale, trans.). New York: Hill and Wang, 1988.

Fee, Elizabeth, and Daniel M. Fox (eds.). *AIDS, The Burden of History.* Berkeley, CA: University of California Press, 1988.

Flemming, Alan F. *et al.* (eds.). *The Global Impact of AIDS.* New York: Alan R. Liss, 1988.

Institute of Medicine, National Academy of Sciences. *Confronting AIDS: Directions for Public Health, Health Care, and Research* (1986) and *Confronting AIDS: Update* (1988). Washington, DC: National Academy Press.

Kaslov, Richard A., and Donald P. Frances (eds.). *The Epidemiology of AIDS, Expression, Occurrence and Control of Human Immunodeficiency Type-1 Infection.* New York: Oxford, 1989.

Koch-Weser, Dieter, and Hannelore Vanderschmidt (eds.). *The Heterosexual Transmission of AIDS in Africa.* Cambridge, MA: ABT Books, 1988.

Kramer, Larry. *Reports from the Holocaust: The Making of an AIDS Activist.* New York: St. Martin's Press, 1989.

Kubler-Ross, Elisabeth. *AIDS, The Ultimate Challenge.* New York: Macmillan, 1987.

Miller, Norman, and Richard C. Rockwell (eds.). *AIDS in Africa: the Social and Political Impact. Studies in African Health and Medicine*, Vol. 10. Lewiston: Edwin Mellen Press, 1988.

Nichols, Eve K., Institute of Medicine, National Academy of Sciences. *Mobilizing Against AIDS.* Rev. ed. Cambridge, MA: Harvard University Press, 1989.

Pierce, Christine, and Donald Van DeVeer (eds.). *AIDS, Ethics and Public Policy.* Belmont, CA: Wadsworth, 1988.

Rogers, David E., and Eli Ginzberg (eds.). *Public and Professional Attitudes Toward AIDS Patients, A National Dilemma.* Cornell University Medical College Fifth Conference on Health Policy. San Francisco: Westview Press, 1989.

Sontag, Susan. *AIDS and Its Metaphors.* New York: Farrar, Straus & Giroux, 1988.

Appendix 2

In Development: AIDS Medicines, Drugs, and Vaccines

The chart below is adapted from information presented by the Pharmaceutical Manufacturers Association in cooperation with the American Foundation for AIDS Research and the Food and Drug Administration. Survey current through February 10, 1990 (dated winter 1990). For updated copies write: The Editor, Aids Medicines in Development, Pharmaceutical Manufacturers Association, 1100 15th St., NW, Washington, D.C. 20005.

ANTIVIRALS

DRUG NAME	UTILIZATION	COMPANY AND DRUG DEVELOPMENT STATUS
AzdU - Azidouridine	AIDS, HIV+ symptomatic, ARC	Triton Biosciences Phase I
BUTYL DNJ Deoxynojirmycin	AIDS, ARC	GD Searle Phase I
CD4-IgG CD4 immunoadhesin	AIDS, ARC	Genentech Phase I
COMPOUND Q GLQ223	AIDS, ARC	Genentech Phase I
CYTOVENE Ganciclovir (oral)	CMV retinitis	Syntex Phase I/II
CYTOVENE (Ganciclovir IV) with Betaseron (Recombinant Human Interferon Beta)	CMV retinitis	Syntex Phase III

ANTIVIRALS, continued

Drug Name	Utilization	Company and Drug Development Status
d4T Didehydrodideoxy- thymidine	AIDS, ARC	Bristol-Meyers- Squibb Phase I/II
ddC Dideooxcytidine	AIDS	Hoffman-LaRoche Phase I/II

ddC
Dideooxcytidine with
  Retrovir
  (AZT)
	AIDS, ARC	Hiscia (Switz.)
		Phase I

ISCADOR	AIDS, ARC	Hiscia, Phase I
PEPTIDE T d-ala-peptide T	AIDS, ARC	Peninsula Labs, Cal Phase I
rCD4 Recombinant Soluble Human CD4	Pediatric HIV infection	Genentech, Cal Phase I
RECEPTIN Recombinant Human T4	AIDS, ARC	Biogen, Mass. Phase I/II
RETROVIR Zidovudine, AZT	AIDS, ARC prophylaxis for all stages & conditions	Burroughs Wellcome Phase I/II
SK&F 106528 Recombinant soluble CD4	HIV+ asymptomatic, symptomatic, ARC	SmithKline Beckman Phase I/II
UENDEX Dextrane Sulfate	HIV+ asymptomatic, symptomatic, AIDS	Ueno Fine Chem, Jap Phase I/II
USHERDEX 8 Dextran Sulfate	HIV infcction, AIDS	Dextran Products Phase I/II
VIDEX Dideoxyinosine, DDI	AIDS, ARC (adult & pediatric)	Bristol-Myers Squib Phase I/II/III
ZOVIRAX Acyclovir	CMV retinitis Herpes zoster	Burroughs Wellcome Phase II/III
ZUVIRAX Acyclovir & Retrovir	AIDS, ARC	Burroughs Wellcome Phase II/III

CYTOKINES

Drug Name	Utilization	Company and Drug Development Status
BETASERON Recombinant Human Interferon Beta	ARC, Kaposi's sarcoma, AIDS	Triton Biosciences Phase II
BETASERON & Retrovir	AIDS, ARC	Triton Biosciences Phases I & III
EPREX Recombinant Human Erythropoietin	Severe anemia associated with AZT therapy	Ortho Pharma., NJ Treatment IND
GM-CSF Granulocyte Colony Macrophage Stimulating Factor with Roferon and Retrovir	Kaposi's sarcoma	Immunex, Wash. Phase I/II
GM-CSF	Leukopenia	Sandoz, Ph. II/III
GM-CSF with Cytovene	CMV Retinitis	Sandoz, Ph. II/III
GM-CSF with Retrovir	AIDS	Sandoz, Ph. II/III
INTERLUKIN-2 with Retrovir	Kaposi's sarcoma	Hoffman-LaRoche Phase I
INTRON Interferon-alpha 2b with Retrovir	AIDS	Schering-Plough Phase II
NEUPOGEN GM-CSF + Retrovir	AIDS, ARC	Amgen, Cal. Phase I
REOFERON-A Interferon alfa-2a with Retrovir	AIDS, ARC	Hoffman-LaRoche Phase II (NIAID trials)
TIMUNOX Thymopentin (TP/5)	HIV infection	Immunobiology, NJ Phase II
WELLFERON Alfa Interferon with Retrovir	HIV, Kaposi's sarcoma	Burroughs Wellcome Phase I/II

IMMUNOMODULATORS

Drug Name	Utilization	Company and Drug Development Status
AS-101	AIDS, ARC	Wyeth-Ayerst, Pa. Phase I/II
AS-101 + Retrovir	AIDS, ARC	Wyeth, Ph. I/II
BROPIRIMINE ABPP	Kaposi's sarcoma	Upjohn, Ph. II
EL10 DHEA	HIV infection	Elan, Ph. I/II
GAMIUNE-N Human Serum Globulin	Pediatric HIV+	Cutter Biological, Phase II/III
GAMINUE-N with Retrovir	AIDS, ARC	Cutter, Ph. II/III
IMUTHOL Diethyldithio- carbamate	HIV+, ARC, AIDS, pediatric	Merieux Inst, Fla. Phases I through III depending upon application
IMUTHOL with Retrovir	AIDS	Merieux, Ph. II/III
LENTINAN b-(1-3)glucan	HIV infection, all phases & pediatric	Lend Chemico, NJ Phase I/II
THYMIC HUMORAL FACTOR	HIV+	Adria Labs, Dublin Phase I

ANTI-INFECTIVES

Drug Name	Utilization	Company and Drug Development Status
566C80	PCP treatment	Burroughs Wellcome Phase I
CILOFUNGIN	Candida esophagitis	Lilly, Ind. approv.
CLINDAMYCIN with Primaquine	PCP treatment	Upjohn, Ph. I/II

ANTI-INFECTIVES, continued

Drug Name	Utilization	Company and Drug Development Status
DAPSONE with NebuPent	PCP prophylaxis	Jacobus Pharm. Phase II/III
DAPSONE with Retrovir	PCP prophylaxis	Jacobus, Ph. III
DARAPRIM Pyrimethamine	Toxoplasmosis prophylaxis	Burroughs Wellcome Phase II
DICLAZURIL	Cryptosporidioisis	Janssen Pharm. Phase I
FIAC Fiactiabine	CMV infection'	Oclassen Pharm. Phase I/II
MYCOSTATIN PASTILLE Nystatin Pastille	Oral candidiasis prevention	Bristol-Myers Phase III
NEBUPENT (see Approved Medicines)	PCP treatment	Orphan drug
NIZORAL Ketoconazole	Candida esophagitis	Janssen Pharm Phase III
ORNIDYL Eflornithine	PCP treatment	Burroughs Wellcome Ind. OK (orphan)
PIRITREXIM	PCP treatment	Burroughs Wellcome Phase I/II
PNEUMOPENT Aerosol Pentamidine Isethionate	PCP prophylaxis	Fisons, Mass. NDA submitted
RIFABUTIN	MAI prophylaxis	Adria Labs, NJ Phase II
SPIRAMYCIN	Cryptosporidial diarrhea	Rhone-Poulenc, NJ Phase II/III
SPORANOX Itraconazole R51211	Cryptococcal meningitis and histoplasmosis maintenance therapy	Janssen Pharm. Phase III

ANTI-INFECTIVES, continued

Drug Name	Utilization	Company and Drug Development Status
TI-23 CMV Monoclonal	CMV infection	Teijin, Tokyo Phase I
TRIMETREXATE with Leukovrin	PCP treatment	Warner-Lambert Treat Ind, Ph. III

VACCINES

Drug Name	Utilization	Company and Drug Development Status
HIVAC-1e	HIV Negative, early infection	Bristol-Myers Phase II
SALK HIV Immunogen	Early HIV infection	Immunization Products, Ph. II/III
VAXSYN HIV-1 (gp160)	Early HIV infection	MicroGeneSys, Ct. Ph. I/II vaccine Ph. I therapeutic

OTHERS

Drug Name	Utilization	Company and Drug Development Status
MEGACE Megestrol Acetate	Anorexia and cachexia treatment	Bristol-Myers Phase II/III
MESALAMINE	Inflammatory Bowel Syndrome	Norwich Eaton Phase I/II
SANDOSTATIN Somatostatin	HIV related diarrhea	Sandoz, Ph. II/III

Index